DIETS
SUCK

THE ULTIMATE BLUEPRINT ON
ENJOYING FOOD AND GETTING LEAN

PRAISE FOR
DIETS SUCK

Josiah is a breath of fresh air in an industry full of deception and snake oil salesmen. The fitness industry needs more honesty and integrity, and Josiah is a part of a movement to bring real truth in fitness education.

Sal Di Stefano
Co-Host of Mind Pump and creator of the MAPS Program

Josiah Novak and his coaching have been invaluable on my path to taking control of my health. With all the self-proclaimed "health gurus" out there, it can be hard to sift through the noise when it comes to what path is right for you. Josiah cuts through the B.S. and gets to the root of the habits, practices, resources, and accountability to get leaner, stronger, and healthier.

Ryan Michler
Author of *Sovereignty*, Owner and Founder of Order of Man

Josiah's honest and simple approach to taking control of your health, nutrition, and lifestyle is exactly what the fitness industry needs. With all the misleading and confusing information that plagues the health industry, Josiah clears a path for you that, if followed, will level up your health and your life.

Adam Schafer

Co-Host of Mind Pump and IFBB Pro Physique Athlete

Josiah Novak is not only a knowledgeable expert when it comes to nutrition and fitness, he genuinely cares about each client and their results. He constantly goes above and beyond to ensure each program is right for his client and ensures they will achieve results. There are a lot of cookie cutter coaches out there. However, Josiah is the real deal!

Larry Hagner

Host of The Dad's Edge Podcast and Owner of The Good Dad Project

When I first met Josiah Novak, I was extremely impressed with his knowledge of fitness, nutrition and the impact he was creating as a coach. Just because you have knowledge does not mean you are going to excel at the art of coaching and this is where Josiah thrives. He is creating massive impact in this world through his coaching his content, his podcast and now with his book Diets Suck.

Tony Stephan

Registered Dietician, and Host of the School of Success Podcast

DIETS SUCK

THE ULTIMATE BLUEPRINT ON ENJOYING FOOD AND GETTING LEAN

JOSIAH NOVAK

Diets Suck: The Ultimate Blueprint on Enjoying Food and Getting Lean

Cover design: Jason Woodrich

Editing: Kathryn DeHoyos

Interior design and typesetting:
Courtney Hudson, Lorenne Marketing & Design

ISBN 978-0-578-40044-0

Printed in the United States of America, First Printing, 2018

DEDICATION

This book is dedicated to my wife Michelle and our two boys —
Jaxson Josiah Novak and Cameron Alexander Novak. Michelle, to put
it simply, I love you. I love that you allow me to be my crazy, creative
and often wild self. Thank you for being such an incredible, unselfish
and caring mother and wife. Your dedication to ensuring our boys are
healthy, loved, and cared for is inspiring.

To Jax and Cam - one day I know you'll read this book and as I wrote
it all I thought about was what you would think. Your opinions are all
that matter to me. As your father, I'll never pretend to know it all, but
I will always strive to learn more each day so that I can teach you and
lay a path for you to follow. Eventually, I hope this book inspires you
both to create your own path and explore this incredible world we
live in. I love you both so much. Thank you for challenging me and
inspiring me to grow as man and father each day.

TABLE OF CONTENTS

04   How to Set Up Your Nutrition Plan. 63

05   Setting Up Your Meal Plan 77

ACKNOWLEDGEMENTS

I'd like to first and foremost thank all the incredible and talented people who helped make this book happen. My editor Kathryn, my team (Jeff, Jordan and Jason), and my fellow fitness professionals who pushed me to get this book out have all made this process incredibly enjoyable. Without you all, this book would never happen.

I'd also like to thank all the amazing and hard-working clients that I've had the pleasure of working with over the past 15 years in the health and fitness industry. Your trust and commitment to working with me have allowed me to accumulate countless hours of experience which has led to the formation of this book. I never take a single client for granted, and I'm so lucky to have had a chance to impact your lives. Whether you know it or not, you've hugely impacted my life.

Finally, I want to thank all the mentors I've had along the way. There's a long list so I've been sure to include them in "People You Should Follow" section of this book. I am humbled and honored to have had such talented and inspiring people in my life who have pushed me to level up both as a professional and as a person. Your knowledge, mentorship, and commitment to helping others have helped me create my dream career. I am eternally grateful, and I pray that one day I'll have the chance to buy every one of you a Moscow Mule.

FOREWORD

Being asked to write the foreword to such an amazing book is an honor. And while I want to ensure that I adequately fulfill what was asked of me, I also want to respect your desire as the reader to get to the book. For that reason, I will be brief and to the point.

Connection is the essence of growth as a human being — and one fateful Sunday night, I walked into Gold's Gym in Chantilly, Virginia and created a connection that will last me a lifetime.

I wish I could remember the date to give you some context, but as of the time of writing this (2018), my best estimation is that it was about ten years ago.

At this time in my life, fitness was everything. My diet was always near perfection, I never missed a workout, and my social circle was small because I only connected with other people that lived a similar lifestyle.

But on this Sunday night, I noticed someone in the gym as I was training ...

He seemed to be about my age, and appeared to be in great shape ...

He was training hard, and not talking to anyone ...

And while I would love to have some magical story around how we began our conversation; the truth is that I don't remember what initially prompted our connection ...

What I do know is this — after ten years of friendship, this is a night that I am forever grateful for!

Somehow, we did end up striking up a conversation, and immediately built a bond that has seen ups, downs, and everything in between.

If you don't know me, my name is Jason Phillips, CEO of iN3 Nutrition and The Nutritional Coaching Institute. And while I mentor a lot of people in this world, I consider Josiah Novak to be one of the best mentors I have ever had and will ever have.

A mentor is someone that understands THE TRUTH, and that is exactly what Josiah has always been there to provide in my life.

He is the one and only friend that attended my one bodybuilding show.

He is the person who supported me when I lost family members.

He is one of the few people in the world who has genuinely been happy to see my success.

But most of all, he is the person I look to as an example as I continue to evolve into the husband, father, and leader I am becoming.

Why do I tell you this? After all, this is a nutrition book not a biography of Josiah ...

The reason I tell you is because you need to understand the character of the man that is leading you.

What you may not realize yet is that your nutritional success is not only dependent on your food choices. It can be dictated by several factors in your life, including the way in which you handle your roles as parent, spouse, and friend.

And while there are a lot of people in this world that have mastered the biology and physiology behind food, very few understand and truly live the lifestyle needed for successful transformation.

This is what Josiah has mastered, and it is the exact reason he has created so many successful TRUE TRANSFORMATIONS.

But here's some more truth — you are not reading this book for Josiah or me — you are reading this book for you.

You are reading this to find the tools necessary to build the body you desire.

With this body will come the self-belief that has been missing for years.

You are reading this to build the self-confidence you have been lacking.

With this confidence, you can become the spouse and partner that you know you are

You are looking to clear up the confusion that clouds your daily food decisions

With clarity comes action — successful action!

Having read this book, I can confidently say that you are not about to read something that will help you change your diet. Instead, you are about to find LIBERATION.

Liberation in choices around your food ...

Liberation from the stories you have told yourself about not being worthy of change ...

And liberation from anything holding you back in your pursuit of successful transformation!

My friend, having personally walked a journey with Josiah for the last ten years, I can tell you that you are in good hands.

Commit, take action, and GO ALL IN on yourself in this journey.

You deserve to have it all, and now you have the resource to make it happen.

Enjoy the ride!

With love,

Jason Phillips

INTRODUCTION

"Resistance cannot be seen, touched, heard or smelled. But it can be felt. We experience it as an energy field radiating from a work-in potential. It's a repelling force. It's negative. Its aim is to shove us away, distract us, prevent us from doing our work."

Steven Pressfield, *The War of Art*

Diets suck. Diets are temporary Band-Aids that end up having to get ripped off and replaced time and time again. If you want a true transformation, you're going to have to kick diets to the curb like that crazy ex that stalks you at the local Starbucks. Reading this book is the first step to ending your relationship with fad diets once and for all.

It's time to tell the truth. If you're a human being and you're reading this right now, my guess is that you want to look good naked. You also want to enjoy some food like tacos and beer, pizza and wine, or ice cream and tequila. Ultimately you don't want to die young because of poor health, and you'd like to feel good when you wake up each day. When it comes to checking the "life and health" boxes most people want to look good, feel good, and perform well each day. If all those boxes are checked you'd be pretty well off when it comes to health, fitness and living the good life.

This book is designed and written to give you the truth about nutrition and how to set up your eating plan for success. This is the book for you if you're looking for a simple, clear and enjoyable plan to look, feel and perform your best.

Before we go forward ... it's important to take a quick look back.

If you don't know me already, my name is Josiah Novak. I'm a health and fitness coach, host of the True Transformation Podcast, writer, owner of TheTrueTransformation.com, and dedicated family man.

Despite having achieved high levels of success in the fitness industry, I've always been very self-conscious about my body. Growing up I was athletic, but very skinny. The only part of my body that wasn't skinny was my stomach. Yep, I had a Dad-bod as a young adolescent.

My relationship with food has never been what I would describe as healthy. I ate whatever I wanted whenever I wanted. Being active throughout most of my life had allowed me to eat fast food, junk foods, snacks and whatever I was craving. All my body fat was around my stomach and my legs, so I didn't appear to be carrying excessive weight. However, I felt super insecure about my body.

Once I hit college, I knew that I needed to get control of my nutrition or else I'd be destined for a lifetime of frustration and insecurity around my body. Despite knowing that I needed to make a change, my bad habits and frustration only continued to get worse.

It's scary to think that at one point I was so depressed and fed up with my pursuit of health and fitness that I almost took my own life. Nothing was working. I couldn't stick to any of the diets that claimed to be the magical solution to fat loss. I desperately wanted to make a change and feel good about food and how I looked, yet everything

I tried was unsustainable. I was constantly either hungry or feeling sick from binge eating. Every diet I followed ended up failing miserably. My life was spinning out of control and I had tried every diet under the sun to try to get into shape, but nothing was working.

Thankfully, that's not where the story ends. Instead, that suicidal young man (me) was able to turn his life around and figure out the nutrition game. It wasn't easy, but the journey and knowledge I've acquired will hopefully inspire you or at least educate you on how to eat for your goals. If you follow the steps outlined in this book, you'll be able to ignore all the fad diets and create a nutrition blueprint for your life.

Raise your hand if you've ever said or felt this way:

> *Ugh. I feel fat. Time to find a new diet. Maybe I'll try juicing or that new raw vegan diet. Or you know what? I'm going to do paleo because then I'll be able to shed this weight quick and still eat real food.*

Have you heard about that new diet that's so popular right now? That one where you don't eat any food after 6 pm? The one where you cut out all carbohydrates on the weekends? The one where you only eat grilled chicken and veggies for 18 days straight? Have you tried it? What about the diet where you only eat proteins and fats? Have you tried the diet where you just count points, and somehow everything works out?

I bet you're reading this thinking, "I've tried a few diets, and I completely suck at sticking to them for any longer than two weeks." You might have tried more than a few. Or maybe you've never tried one, but you've considered it. Either way, you've heard of a few different diets. Each one is claiming to be the latest and greatest cure for weight loss, muscle gain, sex drive, blah, blah blah.

With all of these diets fighting for your attention, you'd think the world would be jam-packed with lean, strong, healthy and fit bodies. All these diets should have cured our weight gain issue by now right? Wrong, very wrong.

The truth is that diets suck. And, they suck because they are all temporary band-aids for a much bigger problem. Each one offers only temporary help. They act like pain killers as they temporarily numb the pain, yet at some point, the root of the pain must be addressed. Diets don't offer a permanent solution, nor do they give you the education needed to understand food and how all this nutrition stuff works.

Before you read any further, I want to admit something. I've tried countless diets. I've honestly tried them all. Not only did I try them all, but I've worked with thousands of clients, and I've seen first-hand what following a diet does (and doesn't do) not only for myself but for the many people I've helped guide on their transformation journey. All diets lead you back to square one. Quick results followed by frustration that you can't maintain them and then the cycle starts over.

My personal journey with health, nutrition, fat loss, muscle gain, and weight gain has been full of ups and downs. I was just like you, chasing the latest and greatest diets, pills, powders, and programs all promising the "secret" to looking awesome with my clothes off, having a lean and strong body, and a host of other hot buttons that had me foaming at the mouth with excitement. Chasing these incredibly attractive results not only caused massive frustration, but I wound up gaining 80 lbs. of body fat in my early twenties. It got so bad that at one point I considered suicide.

As a young man, I faced a huge uphill battle with health, fitness and building strong habits to ensure I'd be living my best life. Fortunately, after over a decade of struggling to gain control of my health and fitness, I was able to put the diet fads and temporary solutions to bed. All the struggles, pain and issues with my nutrition resulted in a strong understanding of what an effective approach to eating looks like.

That's what this book is all about. This book isn't meant to bash all the diets that have come and gone. Instead, I want to educate you on what parts of certain popular diets are good and how you can use them to your advantage. Most importantly I want you to develop a simple, healthy, enjoyable and effective approach to nutrition so that you can have the body, energy, health and performance that you've always wanted. You can stop the endless cycle of trying new diet after new diet and for once feel fully in control of your eating habits.

This book is going to outline the important things you need to know about nutrition plus teach you how to apply them to your unique life and lifestyle. You'll walk away with the tools and information needed to get lean, add muscle, improve your health and feel incredible each day. You'll also be able to block out all the noise from all these diets that do nothing but suck your energy and drive you crazy.

Getting healthy, fit and enjoying your nutrition plan can be a simple process. It won't always be easy, but it shouldn't be complicated. Mastering nutrition will come much easier than you think if you block out the BS and focus on what truly matters. That's what this book is all about.

Before you jump in, I just want to say thank you. Thank you for reading this and for taking the time to make a change to your nutrition and your overall health. This book will serve as the strong foundation you need to have when it comes to the food you put in your body each and every day. Just know, no matter what happens, I'll always have your back. I'll always be here to share my struggles and help you avoid making the same mistakes I've made. If you're ready, I'm ready.

THE TRUTH — WHO IS JOSIAH NOVAK?

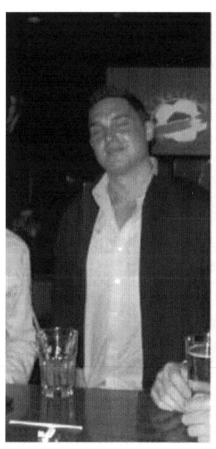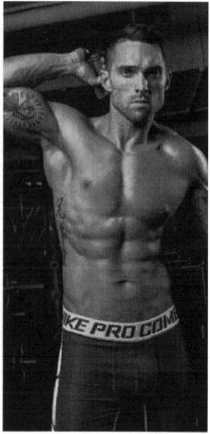

Let me get something out of the way now. I am not a nutritionist, a registered dietician, research junkie or scientist. I don't claim to know it all when it comes to nutrition. In fact, I'm sure I know little in comparison to guys and girls who spend countless hours in a lab finding new nutrition breakthroughs on a weekly basis. I'll most likely never know it all and I'm sure even if I reached that impossible altitude, there'd be new findings that completely throw all past claims out the window.

Here's what I can claim: I'm always learning, and I have years of experience that I'm sure, if nothing else, will teach you what not to do. I am a student first and a teacher second. I believe that continually striving to learn more and prove my theories wrong will ensure that I show up with value for the people I serve. Most of all, I am someone who gives a crap about how to eat and how nutrition and fitness tie into my life and yours. Let's put it this way ... I know enough to be dangerous.

My love for fitness started with hatred. Hatred towards my parents for the turmoil they caused in my house, hatred towards my father who was physically and verbally abusive, hatred towards myself for my lack of confidence, and hatred towards fate for dealing me a bad hand.

I don't recommend starting your fitness journey based off hatred or dislike. As you'll soon see, I ended up paying dearly for this approach.

As a teenager I started working out for 2 reasons. I wanted to get bigger and stronger and I wanted to be able to kick my Dad's ass. I wanted to walk into my high school bigger, faster and stronger so that I wouldn't feel like a small, worthless, insecure dude whose parents were going through a really ugly divorce. Something in my heart told me that working out was my ticket out of the hell that was my house. I was determined to be strong enough to stand up to my father and put an end to the bullying, physical abuse and verbal abuse that I received on a regular basis.

When my high school friend Joel introduced me to Arnold Schwarzenegger my love for weights and fitness began. I remember going to baseball practice and then after getting home I'd jog to the gym and lift weights and then jog home. I had always loved sports, but the gym was something different. I felt truly at home in the gym. It was my refuge and my safe zone. My confidence started to skyrocket, and my body began to change. The feeling of accomplishment that came with training and lifting was something I'd never experienced before.

Growing up I had been skinny with a gut AKA Skinny Fat or SKAT in some bullying circles. Luckily, I had some athletic ability, but I always felt self-conscious about my body. Around the age of 13 I started to develop severe acne. This only added to my already lackluster self-confidence.

My father, despite being an alcoholic and an abuser, was very active and fit. I remember watching him go for runs, do tons of push-ups and pull ups, and live the fitness life. He always seemed larger than life to me as a kid. My mother was also very active. She was highly competitive and ended up winning some races in my youth. This competitive nature was a big part of my decision to go all-in with my love for working out.

As my body began to change, other people started to take notice. In my senior year of high school my new and improved body landed me the nickname of "Juice" — because everyone assumed all my added muscle was because of steroids. Even though I was 100% natural, this nickname gave me a huge sense of pride. There's nothing better than being accused of being on steroids when you're completely natural.

I wasn't lean back then, but I had added quite a bit of muscle and fat which signaled my transition from a boy to a man. My approach to eating during those years was simply "eat as much as humanly possible." I'd wake up, eat a big bowl of Cheerios with whole milk and a glass of orange juice. Then I'd get to school and grab 2 breakfast sandwiches (plus a chocolate milk) from the cafeteria. I'd pack 2 bologna sandwiches with mayo plus I'd buy a school lunch. Our family qualified for a discounted school lunch program, so I'd only pay 50-60 cents for a full meal. By the time lunch was over I'd eaten well over 4000 calories of mostly crap food. I didn't care. I was getting big and strong plus my athletic ability wasn't suffering so I felt invincible. Girls were taking notice and all my peers were asking how I'd done it. Life was good on the surface, but inside I was a wreck. My parents had divorced which left me wondering how my future was going to play out.

After receiving a baseball scholarship, I headed off to a small college near Richmond, VA. My biggest concern going into college was where the gym was, how I'd get enough protein in my daily intake, and how I'd be able to lift and train while playing baseball. I didn't care about which classes I'd take or who I was rooming with. I had received a baseball scholarship, but in the back of my mind, I knew my baseball career would be over soon. Even though I didn't come right out and say it, I had lost my passion for baseball and replaced it with fitness. I remember ordering a book on how professional baseball players train with weights without messing up their bodies and hurting their skills on the field. I was saddened to find out that most players did the bare minimum in the gym to avoid becoming too stiff and muscular. I knew that wouldn't work for me.

I came to a crossroads with baseball and fitness when I suffered a pretty bad rotator cuff injury combined with severe elbow tendonitis. My love for playing the game had reached its peak, and it was all downhill from there. I knew in my gut that I loved working out and being fit, but that my dreams of playing professional baseball were over. Baseball had been my passion for 15 years, and now it was done. For a couple of weeks I felt empty, but that all changed with a new friendship.

One random day as I was lifting in the main campus gym, one of the trainers there approached me and asked if I wanted to jump into a bench press competition they were having. My shoulder and elbow had healed, but I was still hesitant to throw heavy weight around. However, something told me to jump into the competition, so I did. The trainer who had invited me was named Matt and we quickly realized we had a lot in common.

Matt came from a big family just like me and had fallen in love with the fitness game. His father was a pastor and his family sounded like the opposite of mine. They all loved each other and supported one another plus they held a high standard for behavior and devotion to their faith. Matt and I started training together and he suggested I look into working in the campus gym as a trainer like him — so I did. My career as a coach had begun.

Working in the campus gym for almost a year gave me a new identity. People around campus started to recognize me as the "guy who helps run the gym." I met some really cool people there and I found a new confidence in who I was as a person. I quickly realized that I enjoyed not only learning about fitness for my own goals, but also helping people figure out where to start on their personal journey.

After finishing 2 years of college I came to another crossroads. I wasn't on scholarship anymore and I was quickly falling in love with the process of growing my personal training business. Plus, I was broke, and completely stressed out about having to pay for school. I was taking classes that I just didn't find any value in and deep down I knew that I wanted to own my own business. I knew that I needed a change. When Matt suggested I move to the suburbs of Washington DC in Northern VA to work at a large commercial gym with him I agreed right away.

Moving to a new city with one friend, no money, and no clue what I was getting into was definitely a challenge. Training clients from 5AM to 10AM then back at night from 5PM to 9PM was a grind. The money wasn't great because the corporate gym took almost 70% of the revenue before Uncle Sam took his piece. I was making a decent wage but living in the most expensive county in the United States provided some big-time financial challenges.

After training some wealthy people who were in the finance and investment industry, I began to question my choice in career path. I knew I couldn't maintain the schedule plus the money wasn't going to get much better. I had been working with a couple highly successful sales and business minded people who encouraged me to try my hand at sales in different industries. They had given me props for my ability to communicate with people and despite the fact that I didn't look at myself as someone who was great at sales, I decided to jump into sales full time.

Leaving the corporate gym environment was a relief. I could finally get back to just enjoying fitness instead of dreading my work schedule each day. I missed my clients, but something told me that I'd be working with them again in the future.

After jumping around from sales job to sales job I finally landed on, what I thought to be, my life's calling. Life insurance sales. I had a passion for helping people and I knew that health was one of life's most important things. Convincing people to get healthier while protecting their families in the case of disaster sounded like a perfect fit. Plus, starting my own financial planning practice was simple. I was able to obtain my life insurance sales license and start my own business within a couple weeks. Initially it wasn't easy, but I started selling young attorneys and business owners on the fact that they needed to protect their assets, so I started to build traction. Unfortunately, my success was short lived.

When the stock market and housing market tanked in 2009 my business dried up almost overnight. People started cancelling their policies and ducking my calls. I didn't have too many investment clients, but the ones I had were getting out of the market fast. I was just a 22-year-old kid at the time with zero Rolodex and a whole lot of emotional pain that had never been fully addressed. My confidence in my ability to earn a living, build a life and be a man of value began to crumble. I was bleeding money with no idea how I was going to survive.

I went from making a really solid income to losing money fast. My finances took a massive hit as did my self-esteem. I had envisioned becoming a highly successful financial planner who helped everyone protect their loved ones through life insurance and investments but here I was barely able to pay rent every month.

The stress of being broke, losing clients left and right, and having to search for any job I could get started to take its toll. If I'm being 100% honest my eating habits had been really poor at this point for a while. After leaving the gym scene I was so focused on building a career in sales and finances that I neglected to take care of my health. It all caught up to me when I realized my business was failing.

After months of dealing with massive stress I hit rock bottom. I wasn't sure how I was going to recoup all the money I'd lost or the time I felt I had wasted trying to start a financial planning business. I didn't have a strong support system at the time. My friend Matt, who I'd moved to Northern VA with, had gotten married and was starting his family. The few friends I had at the time were all into drinking, drugs and partying their lives away. My fitness friends were all taking steroids and trying to chase the bodybuilding life-style. I felt very much alone. I hadn't talked to my father in years and my Mom was too busy trying to raise my 5 younger brothers and sisters. I had broken up with my girl and at that point I felt like I had nothing to live for. I looked in the mirror and saw a body I was ashamed of. After stepping on the scale and seeing that I'd gained almost 80 lbs I figured that my life was over. For the first time in my life I contemplated suicide.

I had lost my way, but despite flirting with the idea of killing myself, not all hope was lost. Between hours of searching for new jobs on the internet and playing online poker to support myself, I stumbled upon a guy named Greg Plitt.

Greg was a former Army Ranger and had taken over the fitness modeling scene. He was also a motivational speaker and coach who had a website for people looking to change not just their bodies, but their lives and overall mindset. I started watching Greg's free content and a spark was lit inside of me. Greg seemed to have his shit together. The guy was ripped, smart and highly successful with everything in his life. I wanted to have that kind of success. His approach to fitness was all about the mental side of things, and with my current situation this really spoke to me. It finally dawned on me that my feeling of hopelessness was due in large part to the fact that I had neglected my health and fitness. Greg's website was $10 to join so with the little money I had I took a chance and signed up to his membership site.

After watching all his coaching videos and listening to his advice I knew I had a choice to make. Sit around and continue to be miserable or get back to what I knew I loved — health and fitness.

The day I chose to get back in the gym was the day that changed my life forever. It wasn't an overnight success story. Far from it. The early days back in the gym were not pretty. I had gained a lot of weight, so I was really self-conscious, not to mention much weaker than before. But the weight started to come off fast. I focused on making good choices when it came to food and I stayed active outside of the gym. I didn't set a finish line for my goals. I started asking myself, "Can I see myself doing these things and sticking to this routine forever?" If the answer was yes, then I kept at it. If I ever felt like things were unsustainable then I'd back off. Things were improving fast and once again I threw myself into studying nutrition and workout strategies. I landed a stable job as sales representative selling payroll technology. It wasn't my dream job, but it gave me more confidence with financial security and the momentum started to build.

My transformation began in an era that was ruled by bodybuilding magazines and forums. Most of my education at this point was heavily influenced by bodybuilders and fitness models. Naturally I decided to try my hand at bodybuilding to help push myself to lose the unwanted weight.

Arnold Schwarzenegger's "Encyclopedia of Bodybuilding," was the first workout book I ever bought, and it made sense that I'd wind up doing a bodybuilding competition to help get in the best shape of my life. Long story short, doing not one, but two bodybuilding shows wound up teaching me a ton about weight loss and yes, I got into incredible shape. I also realized that prepping for a bodybuilding competition was not sustainable nor was it a healthy way to live. Eating cold chicken, rice and broccoli out of Tupperware every two hours wasn't exactly living the high life. After both of the shows I did, it took an act of Congress for me to stop binge eating. I had lost just about all of my body fat both times, but quickly gained back a significant amount following each event.

After hiring different coaches through the better part of half a decade, the roller coaster ride that was my fitness journey finally started to level off when I stumbled upon the If It Fits Your Macros (IIFYM) approach[1] along with Intermittent Fasting.[2] These two movements truly changed the course of my dietary habits and propelled my understanding of nutrition to new heights.

IIFYM teaches, that so long as you are nailing your macronutrients (protein, carbs and fats), you can eat anything you want. This means that choking down boiled cod and spinach just to stay on the "clean eating" side of nutrition is no longer necessary. You can eat anything you want provided that you nail your nutrient and calorie goals.

Intermittent Fasting says you can skip breakfast and eat big meals at night — both of which felt incredibly natural to me. I was no longer handcuffed by having to either be strict or completely off track. The desire to binge eat slowly decreased as I began eating a wide variety of foods. I must admit my choices in food weren't great back then, but I needed that phase to understand the importance of calories and macros. Fasting gave me a lifestyle that I truly could enjoy. Bigger

---

1   https://www.iifym.com/what-is-iifym/

2   https://leangains.com/the-leangains-guide/

meals at night, the ability to eat out on a date night, and avoiding that dreaded morning post-breakfast sluggishness transformed my entire life. I didn't lose muscle or shrink to nothing, and I wasn't starving. I felt healthier, more focused, and happy that I could structure my nutrition plan around my lifestyle.

I'll always have a special place in my heart for bodybuilding. It taught me many things including how to stay disciplined with my nutrition, that I was capable of reaching huge goals, and that I could improve the way I looked by being consistent with my workouts and eating. However, it just wasn't a sustainable lifestyle. I knew I'd be happier focusing on enjoying a balanced approach versus an extreme competitive sport.

With my bodybuilding days behind me and my new and improved lifestyle — I started to keep the weight off. My confidence started to skyrocket. I was happier, more sure of myself, and I wanted more than ever to start my own fitness company.

Around that time, I was single, but my confidence in my abilities were at an all-time high. I know for a fact that had I continued to really struggle with my self-confidence and my fitness I would have never had the balls to ask my wife out on a date. I actually met my wife at the hair salon where I would get my haircut every 2 weeks. My hair-stylist at the time kept telling me that I had to meet her manager who was also single. The funny part is that my wife's off-day was always on the same day that I would get my haircut, so I would never see her.

Finally, right before my birthday in early October I went on a Thursday to get a haircut instead of my usual Tuesday. When I first saw her, I thought I stood no chance. She was gorgeous and successful. However, my new and improved mindset coupled with my belief in myself drove me to take a chance. I'm glad I did. I'm even

more glad that I told my
wife on our first date that
I wanted to start my own
online fitness coaching
company. She probably
thought I was nuts, but she
supported my dream. She
told me that she wanted to
start a family. I thought she
was crazy too, but some-
thing told me she was *The
One* and the rest is history.

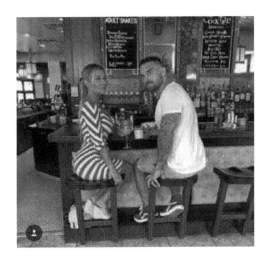

In 2016 I officially quit my full-time job and went all-in with my
coaching company The True Transformation.[3] I had been coaching
and running the business as a side-hustle for about 3 years, but
as things started to grow it got to the point where I had to choose
between corporate America and going all-in on my dreams of
running an online fitness company.

Looking back, there was never a doubt that going full-time with
coaching was the right choice. My company has worked with and
helped thousands of people in the past 5 years. It's been incredible to
see things grow year after year. I always tell people that I'll never stop
learning and growing as a coach and fitness professional.

You can never know it all, especially when it comes to health and
fitness, hence why I'm constantly working to provide the most up
to date and accurate information for my clients and the people who
follow my content.

---

3   https://www.thetruetransformation.com/

This book is my first masterpiece. It will truly change your life if you use the information here and apply it. Nutrition is more than just daily fuel. It's part of our culture, it carries tradition, memories and stories that span many generations.

Food is fun. It tastes great and can bring happiness if used properly.

My goal in writing this book, more than anything else, is for you to have a clear understanding of nutrition and for you to experience the amazing power of True Transformation.

Fitness and nutrition can change your entire life. You can become the person you want to be if you start with taking care of your body and health. Enjoy the book.

01
Diets Suck

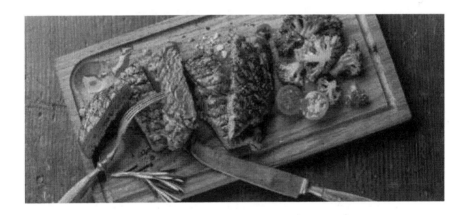

"Fitness is not a sprint or a marathon. It's a lifelong pursuit that has no finish line."

Josiah Novak

FOOD IS NOT THE PROBLEM

Food is amazing. It tastes great. It's part of your culture, your history and it brings back so many memories. The smell and taste of a hot dog at a baseball game, the deep-dish pizza in Chicago, the hot and juicy Kabobs at your local Afghan restaurant, and numerous other amazing experiences are some of the perks of living on this incredible planet. How could you doubt that there's a higher power after biting into a juicy burger and fries on a beautiful fall day?

The problem isn't the food. It's not the New York style pizza that calls your name every time you're in Manhattan. It's not the Friday night frozen yogurt dates with your kids. Food is something you should enjoy.

The problem is, as with anything, that too much of a good thing turns bad quickly. We've taken the enjoyment of food and made it part of our daily routine. Pulling into Starbucks and grabbing a venti, sugar-packed Frappuccino along with a greasy breakfast sandwich once a month isn't an issue. When you start doing that daily — that's when things go sideways.

The world has adopted this "daily reward" mentality which has led to an obesity epidemic that is only getting worse. According to the 2017 Youth Risk Behavior Surveillance System (YRBSS), 14.8 percent of high school students were obese, and an additional 15.6 percent were overweight.[1] The story only gets worse for adults. Worldwide obesity rates have nearly tripled since 1975. In 2016, more than 1.9 billion adults, 18 years and older, were overweight. Of these over 650 million were obese. 39% of adults aged 18 years and over were overweight in 2016, and 13% were obese. Most of the world's population live in countries where overweight and obesity kills more people than underweight. 41 million children under the age of 5 were overweight or obese in 2016. Over 340 million children and adolescents aged 5-19 were overweight or obese in 2016.[2]

---

1   https://stateofobesity.org/data/

2   http://www.who.int/news-room/fact-sheets/detail/obesity-and-overweight

To say these stats are scary would be the understatement of the century. You'd think that with all these diets, cleanses, detox programs and other eating plans that you'd have people thriving instead of dying due to diabetes and other weight-related diseases. What's mind blowing is that things have only gotten worse as the technology and social media age continues to give easier and easier access to information around fitness, nutrition and wellness.

What needs to change? For starters we have to buy into the fact that while we may all share similar traits, each one of our lives has differences. We all come from different environments. We all have different genetics and our bodies all respond differently to foods. We each have unique goals and trying to follow cookie-cutter diets and training programs just won't cut it.

We must stop looking for a one-size-fits-all magic pill and begin to uncover the unique blueprint that will work for you and your incredibly unique lifestyle. This must happen if we want to lead our best lives while also setting up the next generation, who will live in an even more convenience-based society, for success when it comes to their health and enjoyment of life.

The problem we face is our behavioral patterns and the tendency to buy into quick-fix solutions that only serve to create a deeper issue. Diets are marketed as the magical potion that will cure your weight issues and turn you into a fit and sexy human.

Unfortunately, while there are good parts to each diet, without a plan built for you entirely based on you and your life — you will continue to live in the diet, eat whatever you want, gain weight, diet, lose weight, gain weight cycle. But it doesn't have to be that way.

Just by reading this book and investing your time into learning about nutrition you're signaling your desire and readiness to make the lasting changes that will improve the rest of your life.

DIETS ARE NOT THE SOLUTION

The word diet can be used as a noun or a verb. The noun version of the word diet is defined as: *the kinds of food that a person, animal, or community habitually eats or a special course of food to which one restricts oneself, either to lose weight or for medical reasons.*

The verb form of diet is defined as: *to restrict oneself to small amounts or special kinds of food in order to lose weight.* Living restricted is a big stress, not only physically, but mentally as well.

Dieting sucks. Even just the word diet probably makes you feel uneasy. You start to feel trapped and deprived as soon as the word "diet" gets brought up. You picture all the events you can't attend and the amazing food you have to skip out on. You immediately picture a boring life full of boiled chicken breast, iceberg lettuce and mineral water.

The word diet isn't a fun word.

There's a reason why the term "diet" brings on all these negative feelings. You've been conditioned by years of trying all the latest diets only to find yourself back at square one each time. You've felt frustrated, depressed, pissed off, and hopeless when it comes to sticking to a diet. It's no surprise that most people react negatively when they hear the word diet.

Notice how the definitions of the word diet are already a warning sign. *Restriction, restrict oneself, small amounts, special, etc.* If only we'd read the definition before attempting to follow these silly strategies, we'd be much better off.

Unfortunately, we are blinded by our desire for fast, easy, quick and overnight results. Marketers and creators of these diet plans know this all too well. They are fully aware that our natural desires will drive us to not only try their special diet, but also keeps us coming back each time we fail. And failure is just about guaranteed with restrictive diets. Look around next time you're in a crowded space. It's easy to see that weight loss is a challenge for most people.

If diets had a high success rate, we wouldn't be surrounded by obesity.

Diets are strategically designed to prey on your psyche. They sell you on the lie that your weight loss goals aren't being reached due to only one factor. This factor is usually something like too much carbs, too much fat, eating too late at night, eating carbs at the wrong time, eating processed food or eating meat (or not sticking to just meat). It's rather shocking that diets would go as far as blaming one thing for such a complex issue, but it's even more shocking that people continue to believe it time and time again.

Following a restrictive diet can not only be miserable, but it can lead a long-lasting scar that prevents people from wanting to venture back towards improving their health and overall well-being.

Imagine if you tried a few diets and each time you failed miserably. You'd start to think something was wrong with you and that you must not be destined for a lean, strong and healthy body. You'd feel ashamed and guilty because you've convinced yourself that you're simply not good enough, or dedicated enough, or that you lack the skills needed to get in shape. You'd second guess yourself and you'd probably quit trying altogether at some point.

In my book, diets get the "Suck" label for this reason alone. Pushing people away from health and fitness is criminal and it's time to put an end to it once and for all. The last thing the world needs is greater resistance to living a healthy life.

Where did this whole dieting thing start anyway? Would you believe it started as far back as the 1700's? Yep. Dieting has been going on for over 200 years. A Scottish military surgeon named John Rollo,[3] published Notes of a Diabetic Case in 1797. Rollo pushed an "all meat" diet to help treat diabetes. His dietary approach was very successful for treating what we now call Type-2 Diabetes. Funny enough, the all-meat diet craze has recently hit the airwaves again, stirring up all sorts of debate and controversy. Diets are very much like the clothing and shoe styles — they die off and then poke their head up again a few decades later. People continue to believe the hype, yet our problems only get worse.

It's about time we figure out what makes all these diets actually worth a second look. Why are these diets successful (if only for a short while)? Luckily the answer is quite simple. All diets have one main factor in common that will help you build a true lifestyle around a nutrition plan that sticks. It's incredibly simple, so let's crack the code on diets once and for all.

---

3   https://en.wikipedia.org/wiki/John_Rollo

02
The Big Diet Secret

**"If anyone claims to have the perfect diet for everyone —
run away as fast as you can."**

Josiah Novak

Would you believe me if I said that all diets are built on the same
principles? These principles are so simple that if I told you, you might
not believe me. You'd think, "there's no way it can be that easy," but
I swear it's the truth. It's time to draw the curtain back on the heavily
guarded secrets that all diets keep close to the chest.

All diets are based around putting you in a large enough caloric
deficit that you begin losing weight coupled with restricting food
choices to a small menu of healthier items. In simple terms, this
means that all diets are created to help you burn more calories than
you eat while improving your nutrient intake. This way your body
is forced to tap into stored body fat as a source of fuel and eventually you'll lose weight plus you'll only be eating a small variety of
healthier foods which means you'll feel better (at least in the short
term). If you stick to the calorie deficit for an extended period of time
you might even lose a lot of weight.

Each diet that exists or has ever existed is built around these principles.

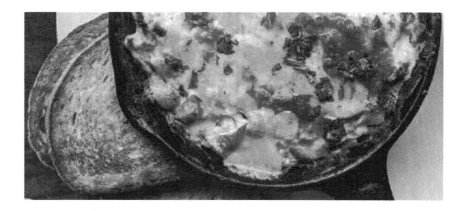

The Keto diet, for example, takes away carbohydrates and tells you to eat mostly fats and some protein. Thus, you can't stuff your face with breads, cereals, cakes, donuts, fried rice and buns anymore. Your calorie intake is going to go down and you'll be eating healthy fats with some protein. Your calories will most likely go down far enough to put you in a calorie deficit and you'll start to lose weight.

You'll blame carbs, but what really happened is that you lowered calories and probably started exercising more which created the need for your body to burn more fuel. All of this adds up to a calorie deficit. You're simply eating less calories than you burn each day and you're getting more healthy fats, so you feel better than when you were shoving all sorts of sugary processed foods down your calorie tunnel (aka your pie hole).

The same is true for any diet out there that causes you to drop fat and tighten up. Whether you stop eating carbs after 6pm or you cut out all junk foods, you're lowering your calories and now your body needs more energy. Your body fat is where the body turns to satisfy this need and your weight starts to fall off. Combine the calorie deficit with improved food choices and voila! Your energy starts to go up and the weight starts to go down.

I'll never forget the day I stumbled upon these incredible truths. I had been trying to "eat clean." That didn't work. Then I tried just cutting my food to barely anything — that backfired quickly.

In my early years as an up and coming coach I had hired numerous fitness "experts" to help me get lean. Each one had a different nutrition strategy. The first one I ever hired told me to cut out all carbs and stick to fats and protein. The next one had me cycling carbs with higher and lower carb days. A couple years later I hired a flexible dieting expert that told me I could eat whatever I wanted as long as I hit my macros. After looking back through my diet plans from each coach I realized that they all had a similar calorie level with a very restrictive variety of food choices. Some of the diets I had followed had been miserable due to the food choices being really limited, but at the end of the day I got super lean following each one. Proper calorie intake coupled with calorie quality was the winning formula. However, one without the other just didn't work.

Making this discovery, for a former overweight and depressed guy like me, felt like I had stumbled upon a cure for world hunger. Ok, maybe not that significant, but it was still one of my most memorable learning experiences. It felt incredible to know that as long as I paid attention to my calories and made mostly healthy food choices I could experiment with a variety of food choices that I both enjoyed and that improved my health (and energy levels).

Each diet that you may see at the top of the popular charts has calorie control as its foundation. Keto, paleo, carb cycling, intermittent fasting, Atkins, and Weight Watchers all are based on controlling your calories. Whether it's cutting carbs out or varying the amounts of carbs and fats you have each day — the number of calories you take in has to be less than what you burn each day if you want to lose body fat. That's the diet secret that all of the most popular diets don't talk about. They'd much rather tell you that carbs are bad or processed food is keeping you fat. I won't argue that the type of calories you eat isn't a huge factor, because it is. However, even if you eat the healthiest food on planet earth, but you don't control how much you eat, you will struggle to get in shape.

As Lou Schuler and Alan Aragon write in their book, *The Lean Muscle Diet*, "if you want to change your weight, in either direction, you must find a way to create an imbalance between the calories you take in and the calories you expend".

Control your caloric intake and you'll control how you look, feel and perform. That's the BIG diet secret. Think about calories as the foundation to a house or the engine in a car. Sure, there's more to it, but we have to get those things right first or else the rest doesn't matter. Now before the diet zealots burn me at the stake, yes, the type of foods and the quality of foods you eat matter significantly. However, if you loaded up on organic, wild-caught, vegan, keto and paleo goodies from your local grocery store and ate healthy all day long yet failed to eat the right number of calories — you wouldn't lose that unwanted body fat and you'd still be at risk for health issues that come with being overweight. When building a house, the details matter. The same is true with nutrition, but without the foundation all the little details will be useless.

Get your calories in line and eat healthy foods most of the time (80-90% of the time) and you'll find that this whole nutrition thing gets much easier. This goes for any nutrition approach. Despite what each diet cult will tell you, these are the two PRIMARY rules that govern our eating.

THE BODYBUILDER DIET

For years the bodybuilding diet dominated the fitness space. Bland chicken, brown rice and broccoli for the majority of your daily nutrition along with the occasional tilapia and sweet potato of course. Talk about miserable right? I remember trying to follow it religiously when I first jumped into health and fitness. The bodybuilding diet consisted of eating 6-8 meals per day every 2 hours (to supposedly ramp up your metabolism and prevent muscle loss — which is complete horse crap).[1] If you simply looked at bodybuilders and their amazing physiques you'd think this was the best approach. We just didn't know any better. Before Facebook, Instagram and the rest of social media — the biggest fitness resources were magazines and online forums. The biggest fitness names were top bodybuilders who, despite being incredibly dedicated (and genetically gifted), were far from "healthy" and trying to follow their diet and routines was a hopeless task and dangerous for most people.

Despite being unsustainable and unrealistic for the majority of people, the bodybuilding diet was the most popular way for people to jump into a weight loss journey. Prepping 6-8 meals a day and lugging Tupperware full of chicken and fish was a public declaration that you were attempting to lose fat and get in great shape. Cardio in the morning and weights at night coupled with a boring, bland and restrictive diet seemed to be the only way to get that flat stomach,

---

1   https://examine.com/nutrition/do-i-need-to-eat-six-times-a-day-to-keep-my-metabolism-high/

ripped abs and toned body that was on top of everyone's fitness wish list.

Despite being the opposite of lifestyle friendly, the bodybuilding diet had some positive attributes. For one, it encouraged eating healthy, whole, nutritious packed foods. Cutting out fast food and sugar-packed snacks was a huge step in the right direction for most people. And since the majority of the population eats around the clock, eating every 2 hours wasn't a hard transition for most. No matter how hungry you were, the next meal was only a couple hours away. That being said, training your body and mind to expect food every 2 hours was a recipe for disaster when it came to appetite control, but we'll cover that later in this book.

Once again, the secret to the bodybuilding diet's success was calorie control. Eating very small portions every 2 hours along with "clean" foods that were very low in calories equaled a plan that enforced the first rule of fat loss — you must eat less calories than you burn in order to lose weight. Plus, when you only have a handful of options (some bodybuilders encouraged sticking to 4-5 foods max) it's very hard to over eat. In fact, when I jumped into a bodybuilding show as a way of motivating myself to lose fat, I quickly became so sick of chicken, fish and the rest of the bodybuilding menu that I literally had to wash down all my meals with a flavored calorie-free beverage like crystal lite or Diet Coke. I got super shredded, but it didn't last long. My unhealthy relationship with food resulted in a temporary trip to lean town, with a quick rebound back to being 30+ lbs over-weight. The bodybuilding diet taught me quite a lot, but the biggest lesson was that it just wasn't sustainable.

Eating the same foods each week (chicken, fish, steak, rice, pota-toes, veggies, egg whites and oatmeal) isn't realistic for most people. Variety is the spice of life and, while I agree that you should stick to healthy nutrient dense foods most of the time, you shouldn't feel trapped and imprisoned by your nutrition plan. The bodybuilding diet, as with any diet, has its pros and cons, but overall it's just very unsustainable for the majority of people looking to create a long-term healthy and fit lifestyle.

THE KETO DIET

The Ketogenic diet, otherwise known as the Keto diet, has gone up and down the popular diet charts over the last few decades. As of the writing of this book, it's currently the flavor of the week in the fitness world. It's become so trendy that fitness marketers are going all-in on its massive popularity and using it as a buzzword in to generate tons of attention. If you're reading this book 20 years from, my guess is that it has come and gone and then come back again. The Keto diet will always be around and that's a great thing. However, it's been touted as a magical diet that turns you into a fat burning machine and, as you'll soon see, that's just not true.

What's the Keto Diet?

Most people think "going Keto" is eliminating all carbs and just eating protein and veggies. This is a common misconception. The Keto diet is primarily a very high fat diet coupled with very low carbs and moderate protein. Roughly 70-80% of your daily calories come from fats coupled with about 20% protein and less than 5% carbohydrates. There are some people who can eat slightly more carbohydrates on the Keto diet and still be in ketosis, but most people find it easier to remain in ketosis by consuming less than 30-50g of carbs per day (mostly from veggies and a small amount of fruit).

Initially the Keto diet garnered lots of attention for its help in treating epilepsy. There's no questioning its incredible benefits in treating epileptic patients.[2]

The primary goal of the Ketogenic diet is to shift your body's primary fuel source from glucose (carbs) to fat. When you lower carbs to extremely low levels and raise fats, the body enters a state known as "ketosis." This is where the liver converts stored fat (triglycerides) into ketones. These ketones become the primary source of fuel for your brain, organs and muscles. This process and shift doesn't happen overnight. Getting into ketosis can take a while. Most people reach true ketosis around the 2-week mark (assuming they stick to the high fat, low carb and moderate protein approach).

The Keto diet is very simple. Eat high amounts of fat, keep your protein moderate (and even low in some cases), and eat virtually zero carbs. On paper, especially for people who are highly intimidated by the thought of following a complicated diet, this seems like the ideal path for someone looking to drop body fat. Switching your primary fuel source from sugar to fat sounds very attractive. After all, if you're looking to drop lots of body fat — you have plenty of fuel to burn. Plus, if you love high fat foods like bacon, steak, eggs, avocado, and nuts — you'll be in high fat heaven. Sticking to this diet sounds rather simple.

As with any diet, there's the initial excitement that comes whenever you feel as if you've stumbled upon the holy grail of fat loss. The Keto diet, I admit, sounds like the perfect way to lose fat and keep it off. How hard can it be to just eat fats and protein (with some veggies thrown in for good measure)? Eating bacon every day sounds

---

2   https://www.ncbi.nlm.nih.gov/pmc/articles/PMC2898565/

amazing and highly sustainable for most people. However, let's take a deeper dive.

The first rule of fat loss still applies to the Keto diet. You must burn more calories than you eat if you want to drop body fat. Unfortunately, in some marketing circles, the Keto diet has been advertised as a diet that's immune to the calorie rules. There have even been programs that claim you don't need to worry about calories when following a Keto diet. This is a flat out lie. Calories always matter. Just because you switch from carbs to ketones doesn't mean calories can go out the window. In fact, since fats contain twice the number of calories as carbs (9 compared to 4 calories per gram) the Keto diet has actually contributed, in some client cases I've worked with, to an increase in daily calories (shocking I know). It's actually not surprising when you break down what people are eating on the Keto diet. Lots of heavy cream, eggs, steak, avocados and bacon can add the calories really fast.

It's important to understand that calories still matter, and the Keto diet isn't a free pass into a fantasy land of zero calorie monitoring.

The Keto diet also puts carbs in the "no-go" zone. If we look at things from an adherence perspective, how realistic is it to assume people will eliminate carbs completely and just stick to fats and protein? Assuming you could get the same level of health and fitness eating carbs in your nutrition plan along with fats and protein, wouldn't it make more sense to have a healthy variety of food options in your routine? Demonizing carbs is also very short-sighted. Completely eliminating carbs and assuming that carbohydrates are the reason you're overweight is completely missing the whole boat.

There's also a whole argument around performance when it comes from going from a carbohydrate-rich diet to a high fat diet. There have been numerous reports of a drop-in performance for people in the gym which can result in lackluster long-term results.

Despite not being a huge fan of Keto as a long-term nutrition approach, I have to admit there are many benefits to utilizing the Keto diet in short term spurts. I go into greater detail in Chapter 5 on how I suggest using the Keto approach, but I'll cover a few points here. For one, going Keto has shown to help tremendously with appetite control. Eating carbs throughout the day causes greater fluctuations in insulin spikes, which can lead to big appetite swings. Controlling your appetite is a huge deal when trying to lose weight. If you're always hungry and thinking about food — it can be a big undertaking when it comes to sticking to your nutrition plan. Personally, I've noticed I have much more focus and mental clarity when going Keto in short spurts. Eventually I miss carbs way too much and, for lifestyle purposes, I go back to a healthy amount of carbs in my diet, but the mental focus and appetite control can't be denied on the Keto diet. The good news is that there's still strategies to get similar benefits without having to go full Keto. I cover these in Chapter 4 and Chapter 5.

The Keto diet also makes things super simple. Having a complicated plan is a recipe for disaster, especially when you're just starting out on a weight loss journey. Stick to fats and protein (with a little bit of veggies) — simple. Simple doesn't mean easy or sustainable, but it definitely takes the guesswork out of things for a lot of people.

When looking at the Keto diet, it's obvious why it's gained such massive popularity. First, eliminating carbs can immediately lower calories for a lot of people. If you go from scarfing down boxes of donuts and pasta to eating a couple eggs and avocados with steak for dinner — you're going to lose weight because you're controlling your calories. Not to mention, most people often experience massive drops in weight when first starting the Keto approach. This is due to your body emptying its glycogen stores and burning through them as you transition into Ketosis. Plus, glycogen stores also contain water and when that glycogen gets used up — the water goes with it. Less water and less glycogen equal a big drop in weight. This initial loss slows down fast and when people add carbs back in its common to see that weight come back on fast. However, for self-belief and mental momentum it can be nice to see that scale number drop when you're first starting out.

The big question you need to be asking with the Keto diet is "can I do this for a long time?" Some people thrive on a Keto approach. Others crash and burn fast. If you enjoy carbohydrates and can tolerate them at a healthy level, there's no requirement to cut them out when it comes to getting in great shape.

If you're highly attracted to the Keto approach, I encourage you to experiment with it. You may find that a high fat program works wonders for you. In fact, I'm a huge fan of a high fat approach for certain days and periods of times throughout your year. I'll go into greater detail in the chapters ahead, but if you're curious about Keto — give it a shot. Just don't buy into the hype that it's a magical pill that doesn't come with rules. The same nutrition rules apply here, just like any other dietary approach.

03
Nutrition 101

"There's never been a time when I've said, 'I really regret working out and training today.'"

Josiah Novak

BUILDING YOUR NUTRITION DREAM HOME

Setting up a nutrition plan is similar to designing your dream home. It's easy to get excited about all the fancy additions or areas you'd like to remodel. The basic foundations can be easily forgotten. This is where most people go wrong.

Getting educated on nutrition is something I recommend everyone not only do but continue to do for as long as they're alive. The truth is that this material should be taught to our children from an early age. Kids are raised in an environment where manufactures deliberately package unhealthy, low-nutrient foods in colorful boxes and place them on shelves at an eye level where kids can easily spot them. Our childhood shapes our beliefs, especially when it comes to nutrition. Most people can name a bunch of fancy diet names, but rarely do they understand how nutrition actually works. It's time to change that.

Imagine hiring a fancy builder to construct your dream home. This builder knows everything about marble floors and winding staircases, yet their resume is lacking a strong understanding of the foundational principles of home building. I highly doubt you'd invest your savings into a builder of that stature.

The same is true for nutrition and eating. You need to first understand the basics and get clear on how food actually works. Only then can you graduate to the fun stuff.

This chapter will give you the basics around what actually matters when it comes to nutrition. I want to simplify things for you and help you easily understand the basic principles that will help guide your nutrition journey.

What I won't do is confuse you with hard-to-understand scientific terminology or bore you to death with the minor details that matter very little in the grand scheme of things. This stuff is meant to be simple and easy to digest so that's what it will be.

THE A WORD

Before we get into the nuts and bolts of calories, macros, proteins, fats, carbs, etc. it's time for me to come clean. I haven't mentioned the most important piece to nutrition. While controlling your calories is the ultimate factor in achieving changes in body composition, there's more to the story.

Diets are built on the calorie controlling principle, yet the success or lack thereof from diets comes down to something called adherence.

The ultimate factor that should come before calories in the ranking of importance is your ability to stick to a plan. The word adherence refers to *your ability to commit to a cause or belief.* In this case, your willingness to stick to a nutrition strategy and commit to that strategy for a lengthy period of time.

If, for example, you are enticed by the low-carb high-fat nutrition lifestyle, but you aren't committed to ditching carbs in favor of fats, your long-term success will be negatively impacted and the chances of you reaching your body and health goals are slim to none.

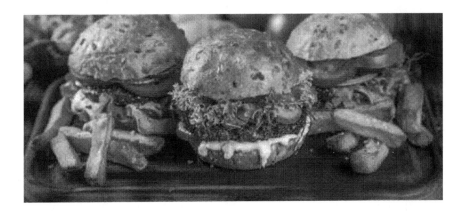

Therefore, before we dive into the basics of nutrition, it's important to remember that learning the science and actually internalizing the information are two completely different things. Our understanding of nutrition is only as great as our ability to use the information given to us, and then apply it to our lives with the full belief and commitment required for success.

Just because we understand navigation, direction, travel and transportation doesn't mean we're committed to traveling around the globe. There must be a firm belief in the plan, yourself, and the tools you'll utilize to achieve your goals if you're looking for long term success with not only nutrition, but anything in life.

In the next chapter we will do a deeper dive on mindset and the importance of self-belief and commitment but understand that adherence to your nutrition set up is a foundational part of eating 101.

In 2008, A to Z Weight Loss study demonstrated the importance of adherence in a 12-month weight loss plan involving obese women.[1] The women were divided into 4 different groups and each group was given different nutrition strategies. Over 12 months, the women who lost the most fat were the ones who reported the highest adherence, despite following different diets. The study concluded that more emphasis should be placed on helping people with adherence versus things like macronutrients and food choices.

Understanding the science behind food is great, but your belief in the plan that can be designed from this science is what will determine your ability to see success. As you learn or review the material in this chapter, be sure to think through how these pieces apply to your life and whether or not you'd be willing to adhere to the principles long term.

CALORIES

Do you know how many calories you consume on average each day? What about over the course of a week? Chances are you may not have any idea how many calories you eat at all. After working with thousands of people all around the world, less than 2% have had a clear

---

1   https://www.ncbi.nlm.nih.gov/pmc/articles/PMC4005268/

picture of how many calories they actually consume each day prior to hiring me. Even the people who I've worked with who claim to have an accurate picture of how much food they eat, after working with me, find that they were actually much less accurate than they originally thought.

A study done in 1992 at the Department of Medicine in St. Luke's-Roosevelt Hospital Center[2] discovered that obese patients who were struggling to lose weight despite claiming to be eating 1200 calories or less (a very restrictive and low-calorie diet) actually were severely underestimating and underreporting their caloric intake. Their conclusion was that the test subjects who struggled to lose weight were not accurately reporting their caloric intake as well as severely overestimating their energy output via exercise.

As human beings, we tend to avoid the realities of our habits and routines. Underestimating our caloric intake is due to both self-preservation as well as a lack of understanding when it comes to caloric amounts. Calorie counting might seem intimidating and exhausting, however once you truly understand the simplicity of calories you'll realize how simple and important it is to be aware (and accurate) when it comes to your caloric intake.

In his book, *The Muscle and Strength Nutrition Pyramid,*[3] Eric Helms lists calories as the most important factor when it comes to nutrition and getting results from your eating plan. With calories being so important, it's imperative that you have a clear understanding of exactly what calories are.

---

2   https://www.ncbi.nlm.nih.gov/pubmed/1454084

3   https://muscleandstrengthpyramids.com/

The definition of a calorie, scientifically speaking, is *the energy needed to raise the temperature of 1 kilogram of water to 1 degree Celsius.* A calorie is simply a measure of heat energy. The term calorie is used to describe how much energy foods contain. A slice of pizza might have 400 calories that your body can either burn right away to help with energy demands or save for future use in the form of body fat or glycogen.

In Tom Venuto's book, *Burn the Fat — Feed the Muscle,*[4] he writes about the Law of Energy Balance when it comes to calories. This law states that to lose weight, you must burn more calories than you consume and to gain weight you must consume more calories than you burn. When it comes to simply losing or gaining weight, this law reigns supreme. However, it's not the only law.

A great analogy for calories is like an organized, well stocked refrigerator full of food. Have you ever gone to the grocery store, bought a bunch of groceries, come home and realized that you already had way too much food jam packed in your refrigerator? You start stuffing things in and moving things around to make space. Things get crowded fast and next thing you know you're considering a bigger refrigerator or an additional freezer to hold all the extra food. This is just like your body. The right number of calories comes with a fit, lean and healthy body (assuming you utilize the calories appropriately). However, eating an excess of calories is like jamming too much food in an already overcrowded space. The only option is for the body to store those extra calories as fat and you'll consistently add weight to accommodate the excess energy intake.

---

4   http://a.co/d/eaNH54K

At this point you might be asking "how many calories should I be eating?" We dive into that in Chapter 4 where I'll outline how to set up your starting plan.

While total calories dictate which direction your weight will go, the type of calories matter too. If your diet consisted of just carbohydrates, even with the right caloric intake for your goals, you'd experience quite a few unwanted health issues, as well as less than ideal results.

In the next chapter we will dive into macronutrients (protein, carbs and fats), all of which contain calories and each one providing different things for the body. There's no denying that calories count, but that's not where the story ends. The type of calories you eat matters too.

MACRONUTRIENTS

Adherence and calories make up the foundation and basic structure of your Nutrition Dream House, but that's not where the story ends. Not all calories are created equal when it comes to your health and fitness. Total calories matter, but where those calories come from is incredibly important as well.

If your body needs 3000 calories per day to maintain your weight and you get all 3000 calories from protein vs. someone else with the same calorie needs that gets all their calories from carbohydrates — you'll be getting 2 completely different results.

A nutrition plan that focuses on proteins, carbs, and fats from healthy sources vs. a plan that gets most of its nutrition from highly processed and greasy fast food, even if the calories are equal, will create two vastly different results in energy, appearance and overall health.

Understanding the importance of calories is the first step in getting control of your nutrition and gaining clarity around why some diets work and some don't. The next step is to understand where calories come from so that you not only lose weight, but you also look good naked, feel awesome when you go about your daily routine and optimize your health so that you live as long as possible (and thrive in the process!).

There are three types of nutrients that make up the foods that you eat. These are protein, carbohydrates and fats. Over the years both carbs and fats have had their fair share of time serving as the villain of nutrition. My prediction is that protein will have its moment in the negative spotlight soon enough.

At the time of this book, the current rage is the ketogenic diet where you eliminate virtually all carbohydrates and focus on fats and protein. If you read chapter 2 you know that eliminating an entire nutrient from your diet is a sneaky way of lowering your calories. However, unless you suffer from a genetic or medical condition that requires the elimination of certain nutrients, having all three macros (protein, carbs and fats) in your plan is a much more sustainable approach.

When it comes to macronutrients, the bottom line is that all foods have a at least one, and sometimes all three, of these macronutrients. Technically speaking — in order to stay alive — you'd only need to consume proteins and fats. These two nutrients are vital for tissue repair, hormonal health, brain function and heart health. However, this doesn't mean that all you should consume are meats, fish, oils and butter. Technically you could live without eating carbohydrates, but carbs have become the go-to source for fuel when it comes to workouts and activity, especially in Western culture.

Carbohydrates are everywhere. Fruits and veggies contain mostly carbohydrates and there's plenty of evidence that having both fruits and vegetables in your nutrition plan will improve your health and overall quality of life.

You'll get introduced to my signature method — "The Power Method" — later in this book, but if you haven't guessed by now I don't recommend eliminating any macronutrients. Most people will thrive off having all three in their nutrition plan. The only exception is for people who are dealing with certain medical or genetic conditions.

Remember, everyone is different, and each person will need slightly different amounts of each macronutrient. We will break down each one in the coming chapters so that you get a better understanding of why each one is important for your goals.

PROTEIN

I love starting a macronutrient discussion with protein. Protein has become the universal nutrient symbol for health fitness. Between protein powders, protein bars and protein "boosted" foods — our culture is in a protein frenzy. I'm sure you won't be shocked to find that the protein hype is a bit overrated, however protein is vital to survival and can have tremendous benefits if utilized properly.

Let's cover the stuff you need to know about protein.

Higher protein diets have consistently been shown to result in greater weight loss, fat loss, and preservation of muscle in comparison to low protein diets. There're a few reasons for this. First, protein is crucial in the muscle-building and muscle-retention process. Protein is also highly satiating which helps control appetite and cravings.

In my personal experience as well as my clients' experience, protein helps tremendously when it comes to feeling satisfied at each meal. This is crucial, especially for someone who struggles with appetite control and hunger.

Protein is the most important nutrient when it comes to muscle creation and maintenance. Protein does more in the body besides build muscle, but its main responsibility is to take care of construction inside the body — both for new tissue and taking care of the current tissue. Your body needs a certain amount of protein to survive. This amount varies from person to person. Once those basic demands are met then additional protein can be utilized to build muscle and improve body composition.

HOW MUCH PROTEIN DO YOU NEED?

The amount of protein needed for your body is a debatable topic, as it depends on both your body weight and activity level. Although there is no set of perfect guidelines, it seems that the scientific consensus has currently landed in the following approximate ranges:[5]

The base level (assuming no activity and no desire to change body composition) is around 0.8g per kilogram body weight (50g for a 137.5lb person) or above. More is not harmful, but this seems to be the bare minimum.

An athlete or highly active person, or a person who is sedentary and looking to lose body fat would do well with a range between 1-1.5g per kilogram. For a 200lb person, this equates to 91-136g daily.

---

5   https://www.bornfitness.com/how-much-protein-do-you-need/

An athlete or active person who wishes to beneficially influence their body composition (lose fat and/or gain muscle) or a very highly active endurance athlete should be consuming in the range of 1.5-2.2g per kilogram daily (for our 200lb person, this equates to 136-200g daily).

THE TYPES OF PROTEIN

There are two types of protein — complete proteins and incomplete proteins. Dietary proteins are made up of about 20 amino acids and complete proteins contain adequate amounts of 9 amino acids that your body must get from outside sources.[6] If a protein source has adequate amounts of all 9 amino acids, it's determined to be a complete protein. This is why foods like chicken, beef, and eggs are popular protein choices. They are made of up of primarily protein (with some fats) and have all 9 essential amino acids.

The 9 amino acids are:

- histidine
- isoleucine
- leucine
- lysine
- methionine
- phenylalanine
- threonine
- tryptophan
- valine

---

6   https://www.bornfitness.com/high-quality-protein/

This is also why I get a good laugh when someone argues that broccoli is an excellent source of protein. While I agree that broccoli is an excellent source of nutrition and that it does have 5g of protein (on average) per serving, unfortunately it's an incomplete protein.

Incomplete proteins are not totally useless when it comes to protein needs in the body. In fact, if you combine foods that on their own are incomplete, but together form a complete protein — you'll give your body the complete amino acid profile that it's looking for.

FATS

It's pretty crazy to think that not that, not long ago, fats were considered the biggest "problem" in our nutrition plan. Back in the 1950's there was a significant portion of middle-aged men dying of heart disease.[7] A scientist named Ansel Keys proposed that saturated fat was causing men to have high cholesterol, which was leading to an increase in heart disease. Keys proposed that saturated fat was the culprit. Funny enough, Keys purposely left out many countries that consumed high amounts of saturated fat but had low rates of heart disease in his studies. This led to the adoption of the low-fat diet approach.

In 2011, the case against Saturated Fat was re-opened and the evidence was shocking. While replacing saturated fat with vegetable oils did lower cholesterol — the studies found that low cholesterol didn't correlate to lower rates of heart disease.[8] Quite the opposite, actually. As subjects lowered their cholesterol — rates of heart

---

7   https://academic.oup.com/jhmas/article/63/2/139/772615

8   https://www.bmj.com/content/353/bmj.i1246

disease actually skyrocketed. The war against fat was over. Fat was officially back on the menu.[9]

For multiple decades people swore by the low-fat diet for weight loss. It's no shocker that people lost weight when they started cutting out dietary fat. Dropping fat from their diet meant less calories — which of course, if you've been paying attention, means weight loss (assuming you're burning more calories than you eat). This of course led to the false belief that scientists who demonized fats must be correct. Yet, as scary as it sounds, scientists get things wrong and their motives aren't always pure.

Hence, why I strongly recommend always doing the research and investing in people who are actually working with people instead of just in a lab. Weight loss doesn't always mean optimal health — as was the case with the low-fat movement.

Fats do many amazing things in the body. Here's a few of their responsibilities:

- Transporting nutrients throughout the body.

- The absorption of vitamins like A, D, E and K in our body.

- Being the structural building blocks for hormones (fertility, sex drive, etc.) and immune function.

- Insulating nerve fibers and transmitting nerve impulses (keeps your brain working).

- Regulating metabolic issues within the body (insulin resistance and diabetes).

---

9   https://www.health.com/health/gallery/0,,20477647,00.html#saturated-fat--0

- Providing a big "bang" of nutrients, turning off hunger signals and eliminating cravings.

It's safe to say that fats are important. In fact, without dietary fats you'd die. Your body literally needs fat to survive. The fact that we ever thought low-fat diets were a good idea is beyond me.

Fats taste amazing and coupled with the fact that a gram of fat equals 9 calories (double that of carbs and protein) — it's easy to quickly add up calories when consuming foods that are high in fats. This doesn't mean you should avoid fats. It's simply a heads up that you should be aware of the fat content in the foods you consume and plan accordingly when it comes to setting up a successful nutrition plan.

FATS YOU SHOULD AVOID

Trans fats, known as fats with partially hydrogenated oil, should be avoided completely. If you read a label that contains "partially hydrogenated vegetable oil" my recommendation is to stay away.

Any type of hydrogenated oils should be avoided as much as possible when it comes to the fats you consume.[10] Alan Aragon, a highly respected expert research scientist in the health and fitness industry, pointed out in one of his research reviews, "Hydrogenation of vegetable oil is a well-established way to [turn] a relatively neutral oil into a threat to cardiovascular health."[11]

When it comes to other fats — such as monounsaturated and polyunsaturated fats — you're going to get health benefits for sure. However,

---

10   https://coconutsandkettlebells.com/good-fats-vs-toxic-fats/

11   http://www.alanaragonblog.com/

that doesn't mean you should start gobbling down loads and loads of extra virgin olive oil, nuts, seeds and avocados. Yes, those foods have tremendous upsides, but they should still be consumed in moderation.

Fats such as butter and coconut oil, in small doses, can help with overall health (and enjoyment of food). The key here is to practice moderation and ensure your food intake matches both your health and physical needs.

Fats should be a staple in your nutrition plan but should be consumed in amounts that fit your specific caloric needs.

Fat Sources

- BEST:
    - Extra Virgin Olive Oil
    - Wild Caught Fish
    - Avocados
    - Nuts (unless you have a nut allergy)

- OCCASIONAL:
    - Butter
    - Coconut Oil
    - Avocado Oil

- RARELY (as close to NEVER as possible):
    - Trans Fats

CARBOHYDRATES

Finally, we get to the section on carbs. I've wanted to write this portion of the book for years simply because over the past decade carbs have become what fats used to be — the main target of blame for our society's weight and health issues. I'm going to cut right to the chase with you here, because this chapter won't be long (but it will be powerful).

CARBS ARE NOT BAD.

Read that again. Say it out loud. Carbs, as with any other nutrient, must be utilized in a way that best fits you and your lifestyle. Too much of anything isn't good for you — that goes for carbs, fats, sex (ok maybe not sex), alcohol, social media, and pretty much anything else.

When you think of carbs do you picture fresh fruits and veggies from your local farmers market? Well you should. Fruits and veggies are carbs. You probably think of donuts, candy bars, breads, pastas, and the typical "carbs are evil" images that Keto Cult members post on a regular basis.

The interesting part is that "evil sugar foods" such as Ice Cream, cake, donuts, and Kit-Kats (my favorite candy bar) are actually made up of a ton of fats along with their sugary goodness.

The problem isn't that carbs are bad or that sugar is evil. The real issue is that we don't prioritize carbohydrates (or fats) that serve both our body and health goals. Western society tends to over consume fried foods along with loads of sugar which is highly detrimental to overall health. Coupled with a lack of exercise and activity, you're looking at a recipe for disaster (pun intended).

Carbohydrates are just the most recent nutrient to take the fall for our lack of accountability around weight loss and health. My prediction is that protein is next in line for the chopping block. Mark my words, at some point in the future protein will be considered evil and all these "protein boosted foods" will be the target when it comes to fixing our health issues.

It's a shame that people are so short sighted when the reality is we tend to simply over-eat foods that taste good because of emotional, stress management, mental and physical issues that need to be addressed. Our issue isn't carbs. It's how we use them.

EATING CARBS RESPONSIBLY

If you're active, workout on a regular basis and tend to move a lot throughout the day — chances are that you'll be able to eat and process a higher amount of carbs in your nutrition plan. If you're very sedentary, workout infrequently or are carrying a lot of excess body fat — you'll probably need less carbs.

These are general rules and there's going to be exceptions of course.

My number one rule for carb consumption is to ensure that you're getting plenty of vital nutrients from fruits and veggies.

Some of my clients get just about all their carbs from fruits and veggies simply because they feel better and see better results with this approach. Other clients include moderate amounts of starchy carbs such as potatoes, rice, quinoa and whole wheat pasta. There are other clients who also include breads, oatmeal, wraps, and the occasional small amounts of candy to satisfy their sweet tooth.

Carb intake and choice of carb type comes down to your individual needs. In chapter 4 I'll give you more specific suggestions around how many carbs you should be taking in based off your goals but remember that everyone is different.

Carb tolerance varies from person to person. For example, I was always told that oatmeal was super healthy yet every time I included oatmeal in my daily meals I felt like death for hours after. The digestion just didn't agree with me and my body. Once I cut out oatmeal and replaced it with fruit I felt 10x better. This doesn't mean that oatmeal is bad for everyone, but it just didn't work well for me.

Sugar, which is a form of carbohydrate, has really taken on the role as the evil villain in the nutrition world as of late. However, just saying that sugar is bad for you is way too general a statement. Refined sugar and high fructose corn syrup, 2 types of sugars, have been linked to higher probabilities of diabetes, insulin resistance and obesity so it makes logical sense to avoid foods that contain them.[12] However, fruit contains fructose, another form of sugar, which is processed by the liver and won't lead to poor health if consumed in proper amounts.

This is where it's incredibly important to understand the context of advice and nutritional recommendations you see online. Recently there was a big name on YouTube who came out and said that eating bananas are the same thing as eating Reese's cups. His claim was that the nutrition you get from a banana could easily be replaced with a greens powder he was selling and, in the process, you'd avoid all the sugar that bananas contain. His comparison of bananas to Reese's cups immediately signaled that he was simply trying to sell you his products instead of educating the public on the truth about bananas. Bananas have nowhere near the nutritional makeup of a Reese's cup, but since they contain sugar they are on the chopping block for marketers looking to scare you into buying their products. Sugar today is what fat was 20 years ago.

---

12   https://www.bornfitness.com/do-carbs-make-you-fat/

The final word on carbs is that everyone needs a different amount along with different types depending on where they are now, their lifestyle, workout schedule and digestive health.

The best place to start is with fruits and veggies (emphasis on the veggies) and then feel free to add more starchy carbs as you assess your tolerance.

04

How to Set Up Your Nutrition Plan

"Even a cowboy falls off his horse at times. He still gets up, dusts himself off and keeps riding. When you fall off your nutrition and workout plan, don't give up. Get up and keep riding — you're still a cowboy."

Josiah Novak

Most nutrition plans and diets completely leave out the mental side of nutrition. There's definitely an argument for the mental side being the most important piece. Where you are mentally today is the biggest factor when it comes to sticking to a nutrition plan.

In this chapter we will break down the mental approach that I suggest whenever you attempt to build a nutrition plan that works for you and helps you reach your goals. If you only read one chapter of this book, I suggest you pick this one.

We'll also cover practical tips when it comes to setting up the nuts and bolts of your eating strategy. I'll give caloric starting points that are simple and easy to understand. Coupled with suggested nutrient breakdowns, you'll be armed with a great place to kick off your nutrition plan.

These are simply starting points and of course will need to be adjusted for you individually.

If you'd prefer to have me and my team handle this for you — I recommend you set up a consultation so that we can map out a plan that makes sense for you and your lifestyle. You can apply for a call on my website, www.TheTrueTransformation.com.

TAKE OWNERSHIP

Taking ownership for where you are right now is the fastest way to take full control of not only your life, but your approach to nutrition and fitness in general.

As a society we tend to blame outside factors for most of our problems. We blame our genetics, the way we were raised, a stressful work environment and the friends and family members that influence us to stick to bad habits. While these factors contribute to your well-being, they are not the reason for where you are now. You can't allow factors such as genetics or the fact that your parents got a divorce to control your health and fitness. That's like allowing highway traffic to determine whether or not you're a good driver. Bumper to bumper traffic blows, but it doesn't mean you should plow through the car in front of you or drive like a jerk simply due to the conditions.

You are where you are because of the choices you've made. That's a fact. The good news is that you have the power to make a change. If you're not happy with your current state, it's on you to change that. The faster you can realize this, the faster you can make a change.

If you allow outside circumstances and external factors to dictate your thought process, you'll stay stuck in the cyclical habit of blaming other things for your entire life. This is a huge reason why people never change. They lie to themselves and dwell in self-pity. The life they have, according to them, is due to bad luck, a poor upbringing, and lackluster opportunities. This is just flat out wrong.

Being overweight forced me to get real and raw with myself. I blamed so many things for my physical state. My crappy job, my bleak finances, and my crappy genetics. All of that was me just lying to myself to make myself feel better for my inability to commit to making a change.

Change isn't easy and it's so much easier to lie to yourself and give yourself excuses for staying in the same spot. When you take ownership for your life, health and fitness you take the power back and you're no longer held back by your limiting beliefs. You go from a victim mindset to a champion mindset. This is where the magic happens.

Before you jump into a transformation plan, you need to get clear on the fact that your life and where you are is 100% your responsibility. This step isn't optional. If you attempt to change but you're stuck on this belief that you're not entirely responsible and that there are many other factors that hold you back and keep you from reach your goals, you'll be destined for failure. You'll blame your lack of dietary adherence on your job, your kids or your lack of motivation (as if motivation forgot to show up at your doorstep). This is the fastest way to remain the same.

I hesitated to write this chapter because I know it might piss you off. However, if you get pissed off I'm actually quite happy. Change isn't easy. Change is difficult. This book wouldn't be necessary if change was something that came naturally. Our brains want to trick us into chilling out and not doing much since that's typically how we survived throughout our history as human beings. I could have lied to you and said this process will be incredibly easy. Just hit your calories and smile! Yeah right. I wish. This is much deeper.

Diets exist because we want shortcuts. We want to get the most for the least. You want champagne on a beer budget as my friend (and incredible author), Carlton Mack, always says. Ownership is the last thing anyone wants to take. That makes the pain of remaining the same very real. However, the pain must be acknowledged. The pain of owning up to your habits and the way you live your life must be faced. Then you must accept the pain of change.

Actually, you need to chase the pain of change. Confront that shit head on and relish in the pain of creating a new and improved version of you. I promise you that the moment you say, "I'm 100% responsible for where I am and where I'm going," your life will change.

THE 4 PILLARS OF TRANSFORMATION

Don't worry, we're making our way to the actual nutrition details that you'll utilize to get in the best shape of your life and stay there. However, I promised this book would make a drastic difference in your life and I must keep that promise. Hence why I'm committed to the truth about Transformation. *True Transformation* is the name of my brand for a reason. It's based on the truth, which is that transforming your life, body and future is difficult. Nothing great ever comes easy and physical transformation is no different.

This leads me to the 4 Pillars of Transformation. When looking at setting up a plan that fits into your lifestyle there are 4 main areas you should be focused on. These 4 "pillars" are meant to create a strong and stable foundation as you go through the process of truly transforming your health, fitness and overall lifestyle.

No plan is safe without a stable foundation. All areas of your life that are of importance to you should be built on a foundation that is rock solid. If you were building a mansion you wouldn't skip the foundation, no matter how enticing all the upgrades and marble floors are.

The 4 Pillars are *Lift, Life, Love and Legacy.* These are the 4 areas we must address when it comes to ensuring your nutrition and fitness plan will stand the test of time. Otherwise, you're going to be stuck in the habit of making progress, quitting, backtracking and having to start over time and time again.

Get these 4 pillars right and you'll dominate your nutrition plan, fitness routine and your entire life.

LIFT

The word lift automatically takes your brain to a workout routine, right? Well, in this case I'm not talking squats and deadlifts. I'm talking about taking your life to new levels.

Lifting your mind, body and spirit to new heights is something that most never experience. The power of improving your health when it comes to leveling up in all areas of life can't be ignored. A healthy and fit person automatically has an advantage when it comes to so many areas including finances, marriage, relationships, sex, reproduction, lifespan and competition.

I will go to the grave with the belief that the fastest way to improve and lift your life up is to get in better shape.

When starting a nutrition plan, or overall body transformation plan, it's imperative that you take a look at the parts of your life that you want to take to a new level. Are your energy and passion suffering? How will a healthy mind and body lift those areas to new levels?

Maybe it's your sex life. It could be your self-confidence. The areas in your life that need to be leveled up will be greatly improved as you improve your health and fitness.

Exercise gives you a natural high from the rush of endorphins that happens after an awesome workout. Over time you'll notice a tremendous lift in natural energy and positive vibes simply by working out and eating well. The feeling of waking up knowing that you stuck to your plan the day before and that this new day is another opportunity to get better is a feeling that can't be matched. Your life will start to transform and the people around you will feel lifted up by your positive energy.

A highly productive mental exercise I use, and I have my clients use is to write down the areas of your life that you want to take to new levels. Maybe it's your relationship with your spouse or it might be your energy around your kids. Are you feeling like absolute shit at the end of the day? Do you wake up feeling like a dark cloud is hanging over your head? As you move to a healthier lifestyle these areas will improve and become strong areas of your life versus areas that are weak.

LIFE

Have you ever sat down and mapped out how you want to live your life? What do you want to accomplish? How do you envision your life playing out? This can be a sobering exercise if you're in a current state of unhappiness fueled by an unhealthy lifestyle.

Life can seem pretty bleak when you feel uncomfortable in your own skin and have zero drive to do anything due to poor energy and nutrition.

Getting in shape won't be easy but mapping out how changing your body and health will change your life is a step that most miss. Blindly jumping into a diet because Jenny in marketing is doing an extreme diet and it sounds like she's getting fast results is not a recipe for long-term success. Your college buddy Chad got abs doing a 17-day cleanse, so you figure why the hell wouldn't it work for you. Yet you have no idea WHY you're doing anything at all. Yes, you know you need to lose weight, but what's life going to look like during your transformation and after you reach your goal?

This whole "being healthy and fit" thing isn't a 90-day process. This has to be adopted into your lifestyle permanently. Mapping out a vision for how you want to live life is a crucial action item as you build the foundation for a successful (and permanent) transformation.

When I finally transformed my body and lifestyle permanently — and found a routine that I could follow forever — it was due the power of visualizing my life. I knew I wanted to marry the woman of my dreams and travel the world while feeling incredible about how I looked and felt. I wanted to be a shining example of health and fitness for thousands of people. I knew that I felt super insecure about the life I was living and the body I was trapped in.

Improving my health and fitness gave me the confidence to ask my wife on a date. Years prior I would have shit my pants just thinking about going on a date with her. I literally told my wife on our first date that I would be a fitness professional and help thousands of people transform their lives. She thought I was crazy at first, but when she saw that I had powerful beliefs around how I wanted to design my life she bought into my plan. What's truly incredible is that the vision I had for my life and the reasons I had for wanting to gain full control over my health and fitness drove me to actually accomplish the goals I had.

I literally married the woman of my dreams and created a fitness company that has and continues to help thousands of people. My fitness routine and the way I approach nutrition gave me the energy to accomplish the goals I had set for myself. It's no accident that my life continues to improve day by day.

I can't encourage you enough to map out your life. Don't be afraid to dream BIG. Put goals in place and create powerful why's for transforming your health and fitness. Your life plan should get you super excited otherwise it needs to be re-drafted until it inspires you to take big action.

Don't skip this step.

You've pinpointed the areas that need to be lifted up and now you will have a detailed vision of how your life will play out. These first 2 pillars are vital to your long-term success.

LOVE

Who do you love? Do you love yourself? These are powerful questions to ask yourself. The love we have for others and the desire to provide security and support for them can be a powerful motivator. However, we can't forget that loving ourselves is just as, if not more, important when it comes to true transformation.

Typically, I see people working out and starving themselves out of guilt and hatred towards themselves. They feel guilty about their lack of consistency and poor habits, so they treat the gym as a punishment and they follow highly restrictive diets to compensate for their lack of self-control. If you were to ask yourself this question: "Would you treat the person you love the most the way you treat yourself?" — what would your answer look like?

Love is one of the 4 pillars due to the power it has in how we approach anything in life. Doing things out of love will translate to more success versus doing things out of hatred. Psychologically speaking, if you're constantly mistreating your body and beating yourself up mentally it's only a matter of time before your body rebels.[1] However, if you do things out of love, even if they aren't easy, you'll find that your success rate improves dramatically.

When I went through the massive transformation of losing 80 lbs. of fat, my initial approach was to punish myself. I truly hated how I looked, felt and performed. I was sick of feeling self-conscious about everything and I wanted to make sure I never went back to my old self again.

---

1   https://www.ncbi.nlm.nih.gov/pmc/articles/PMC2738337/

Unfortunately, I spent quite a few years treating my body like it was my worst enemy. I'd do hours of workouts and cardio coupled with extremely low-calorie meal plans. I lived in a constant state of hunger simply because I was disgusted with myself. I hated who I'd become. Of course, this approach didn't last long. My body rebelled, and I had many periods of time where I'd gain back a lot of the weight I'd lost simply because my body didn't like being abused. It wasn't until I started appreciating myself and the hard work I was willing to do that I began to see lasting results.

Loving one another is important. Yet we can't forget to show ourselves the love we deserve to ensure that we serve others at our max capacity. There are plenty of people who spend their whole lives trying to please everyone but hide their disdain for themselves. Anthony Bordain comes to mind when I think of someone who created so much value and served so many people, yet kept his depression and unhappiness hidden from the world. He ended his own life due to his unbearable unhappiness with himself and his life. If he'd had the support and help he needed maybe there's a chance that he'd have taken a different path.

Love, both for self and for others, is a necessity for life.

Health and fitness are the lowest hanging fruits when it comes to showing yourself love and caring for the body you've been given. This doesn't mean that lifting weights and doing cardio are the only expressions of self-love. My advice is to utilize all aspects of health and fitness when creating a plan to care for yourself.

Yoga, massage therapy, meditation, walking, swimming, paddle boarding, and many other forms of fitness all should be utilized in our quest to treat ourselves with the utmost care. Coupled with healthy nutrition, quality sleep and relaxation — you have a powerful formula for self-love.

This can then be translated into showing the people around you how much you care with the unconditional love that we all have the capacity for giving to the world and our loved ones.

My love for my wife and children allows me the privilege of taking a bullet for them without a moment's hesitation. This unconditional love only grows stronger by my ability to show the fuck up every day for them. I'm far from perfect. Sometimes I still find myself thinking hateful thoughts about who I am in certain moments. I lose my cool or lack patience in certain situations. However, my health and fitness routine bring me back to a place of love. A place where perfection doesn't exist. Instead it's simply progress. Daily rituals that fill my cup and give me the physical, mental, social, and spiritual resources necessary to love those who I care for deeply.

Your transformation will stand strong as you build a foundation around the love you have for yourself and the people you care about. Your routines and the habits you create should build you up and allow you to be the amazing person that you truly are to the people who need you the most.

Notice that love has nothing to do with the diet protocol you follow or the workout routine you choose. Love yourself and decide on the best plans from a place of healing — instead of picking the options that will cause the most pain.

LEGACY

The word legacy, for me at least, always brought on thoughts of dying and leaving behind memories that would stand the test of time. And while I won't deny that leaving the world a better place is a huge part of legacy, I'd argue that what we do while we're here matters even more.

The people we impact, the strong and positive paths we forge, and the example of living that we set for our families, friends and loved ones can't be undervalued. This requires being present in the moments we have instead of always worrying about how things will be when we're gone.

Legacy, as I see it, is both how we live now and the standards we set along with the lasting impact we create when our time is up. Living a healthy and fit lifestyle allows us to become assets for the people in our lives instead of liabilities that can devastate families and wreck entire generations. There have been many health crises' that have wiped out lifetimes of hard work along with creating unimaginable stress for the families involved.

Eating is more than just fuel for workouts or to help you look a certain way. Meals shared over deep conversations and intimate connections adds to your life's legacy. The stories and pastimes you create as you break bread with people you care about are memories that will live forever. Food becomes associated with feelings. I tend to associate certain foods or drinks with specific memories of certain people that have impacted my life on a deep level. Burgers in Vegas with my boys. Coffee with my business mentor Jason Phillips. Sushi with my wife the first time we said, "I love you." Taco Bell, while being pretty unhealthy, always reminds me of the journey and struggle I've gone through to get to this point. Guacamole reminds me of my sister-in-law who is such an amazing help with my kids.

Food adds to our legacy. If we abuse it, it becomes a drain on the person we should be. However, you can use the amazing power of healthy relationship with food to impact those around you.

If this sounds crazy, I'm glad. In a world that is all about the status quo, blending in and following the pack, I want this message to sound a little nuts. Legacies that stand the test of time are built through the drive to be different. The discipline to be you and to stand for something different.

My nutrition journey and the lessons I've learned are part of my legacy. The life lessons that I've been given through my endless education around how to eat will add to the teachings I give my boys and the curriculum I share with you.

Fitness isn't just about looking good. Fitness is one of the foundations to leaving a legacy.

THE 4 PILLARS: FINAL THOUGHTS

As you build a fitness routine that serves you and your life, I want you to think about these 4 pillars. How will your health and fitness routine allow you to show up big time in these 4 areas? If your fitness plan only takes away from your life instead of adding to it, is it really a good plan? Of course not! This is why I stand by my opinion that restrictive diets suck, especially long term. Unsustainable plans won't make your life better. Instead they take your energy and prevent you from living the life you were meant to live.

You can have the body you want and the life you want if you get a roadmap that makes sense for you and your lifestyle. If you're ready to get help with this from me and my team, visit http://www.thetru-etransformation.com/Coaching-Application/.

05
Setting Up Your Meal Plan

"Fitness is the number one tool to level up, change your life, enhance your abilities, and create a legacy that will last forever."

Josiah Novak

Meal plans sold by themselves are, for the most part, a complete waste of your time and money. However, meal plans are a great tool to get a clear roadmap for your nutrition plan. They can give you a visual plan, which is a tremendous benefit when just starting a healthier lifestyle.

In this section I'm going to help outline how to set up your meal plan starting with a basic step that most people skip.

The first step, which is usually ignored, is getting clear on what types of food you're actually going to enjoy eating. Imagine a meal plan full of foods that you despise. If you have to choke down your food at each meal your likelihood of sticking with the plan is slim to none.

This is why a template meal plan that's built for millions of people is a waste of your time. Unless that meal plan is full of foods you love, you'll quickly grow sick of eating foods you hate.

I've included a full grocery list in the resources section of my website to help you get clear on which foods to build your plan around. I suggest starting with choosing your protein sources along with your veggie and fruit choices. These are the healthiest and most nutrient dense foods in your plan so getting clear on which ones you'll be eating is a great first step. Then filling in your meals with your carbohydrate and fat sources comes next.

Be sure that the majority of your food choices (80-90%) come from 1-ingredient foods. For example, broccoli is broccoli and salmon is salmon. These are 1 ingredient foods. A cereal bar or protein bar has 10-15 ingredients and can cause some digestion and potential appetite control issues. These foods aren't off limits but shouldn't make up a huge majority of your food choices.

Once you decide on the actual foods in your plan it's time to get a look at your hunger patterns and when you're going to have time to eat.

For the longest time we were told breakfast was the most important meal of the day. This "law" was, shockingly enough, heavily supported by large manufactures of breakfast cereals, pop-tarts, and other cheap processed food. Commercials directed at children with cartoons would remind us to kick off the day with a heavy breakfast to ensure we got our "most important meal of the day" in. This was a lie. The work breakfast, when split into two words, is simply *break fast* — which refers to the meal that you start eating after not eating for an extended period of time.

Eating an early morning meal is simply meal 1 of however many meals you'll consume that day. There is no "most important" meal of the day. All meals are equally important when trying to reach a health or fitness goal.

In Chapter 7 I'll go deeper into why I personally skip breakfast and why it could be a useful tool for you to utilize.

When it comes to meals, I suggest you eat when you have the time and when you're the hungriest. This doesn't mean eating anytime you feel bored, lazy, stressed, tired or pissed off. Usually following our emotional cues is a bad idea when it comes to eating. Not eating when you're bored, feeling tired or overly stressed is typically a better idea.

However, if you know that at night you're usually mentally exhausted and crave a large meal, then it makes perfect sense to incorporate a large meal that satisfies your needs at that time while keeping you on point with your goals. This is just one more reason why cookie cutter diets suck. They don't account for your lifestyle and the typical life events that can cause you to fall off track if you're not equipped to handle them.

A meal plan that calls for you to eat every 2 hours yet doesn't account for the fact that you're super busy and can only eat once or twice during the day is doomed to fail. By trying to comply to that routine you'll end up feeling like a complete and total failure and you'll likely give in to your old habits of eating whatever you want.

Typically, my clients have found the most success when eating 3-4 times per day. This could be set up in a few different ways. First, it could be a morning, mid-day, and evening meal coupled with a smoothie. You could also have a smoothie as your first meal and then a standard meal for lunch followed by a small meal in the afternoon and a large meal at night.

There's no right or wrong here. If you want to get more detailed it probably makes the most sense to have the majority of your carbohydrates in the meal following your workout. Spreading out your protein evenly amongst your 3-4 meals usually makes the most sense as well.

However, don't worry about these things until you've mastered eating the right amounts of food each day and staying consistent with your nutrition intake.

YOUR CALORIES AND MACROS

Let's talk numbers. Whether or not you've tracked calories and macros in the past, your body is always tracking them. The body will always do what's best for your survival — which means insuring that it's using the calories and nutrients you feed it as optimally as it possibly can. No matter what anyone ever tells you, calories matter.

Calories aren't the only factor of course, but they are very important.

This section might get a lot of hate from "experts" and I'm completely fine with that. There are formulas out there that claim to be the "most accurate" for figuring out how many calories you need to eat. Those formulas work really well, but there's one massive problem with them. They don't take into account how many calories you've been eating. They don't know that you go days with very little calories and then have an all-out binge for a whole weekend. These formulas simply give you an estimate disguised as a precise target.

Let me be clear with you. The suggestions I give you in this section are simply estimates and an educated guess on where you should start with your calories and macronutrients. You won't know if these numbers work well for you until you actually try them. Once you're consistent with tracking and monitoring how your body adjusts to these numbers, then you'll be able to manipulate your calories and macros to fit your goals.

Most people reading this want to lose fat. They might say "I want to lose weight" but in reality, they just want to look and feel better. If the scale stopped working tomorrow, yet you looked in the mirror and loved what you saw — would you even care? The numbers we discuss first will be for fat loss simply because I know that's what most people are looking for. We will address muscle/weight gain as well, but let's start with fat loss.

FAT LOSS

I'm going to save you the headache of dealing with complicated formulas and calculators that are out there. They all end up coming back with similar starting calorie numbers anyway, so don't worry about them. In fact, most of them tend to give you higher calorie numbers than you actually need.

Based off my experience the best place to start with figuring out how many calories you to need to start losing bodyfat is taking your goal bodyweight and multiplying that number by 12. For example, if you currently weigh 250 lbs. and you want to reach 200 lbs. — your starting calories would be 2400.

To some of you this might seem high and to others this might seem low. The good news is this is just the starting point. You may need to lower calories or even raise them if you're not seeing good results or if your energy suffers.

Calorie and protein intake are the two main numbers you'll want to consistently hit each day. Carbs and fats can be increased or decreased based off your personal preference.

SETTING UP YOUR PROTEIN INTAKE

Once again, we will keep things simple with protein. For protein you will simply take your target bodyweight and multiply that number x 1. That will be your protein goal in grams for the duration of this program.

If you are aiming for a weight of 200 lbs. — your protein intake will be 200g. As long as you're getting between .7-1g of protein per pound of lean body mass (everything on your body except body fat) you are good to go.[1] Protein intake should remain relatively stable most of the time.

Each gram of protein equals 4 calories. So, for this example, if you were eating 200g of protein per day you'd be eating 800 calories from protein.

---

1   https://www.ncbi.nlm.nih.gov/pubmed/22150425

HOW TO SET YOUR FAT GOAL

The lowest I'd ever recommend someone go with their fat intake is 25% of total calories. Any lower than that and you're risking a negative impact on hormonal balance as well as general health.

Take your daily calorie goal and multiply that number by .25. This will give you your minimum total calories from fats that you'll aim for each day. Take that number and divide by 9 and that gives you your total grams of fat per day.

For example:
- 2400 x .25 = 600
- 600 divided by 9 = 66g

Round this number to the nearest multiple of 5 to keep it easy. So, in this example you'll aim for 65g of fat.

Remember, after you've set your calories and protein – it's totally up to you to decide how to divide up the remaining calories amongst carbs and fats. Also, you don't have to eat the same amount of carbs and fats each day. You can lower carbs on active rest days and increase fats. On training days, you can increase carbs and lower fats. The choice is yours.

Base your decisions on how your body feels, and what you need at that particular time.

HOW TO SET YOUR CARB INTAKE

By now you've set your protein goal and your fat goal, so the calories remaining will be dedicated to your carb intake. Let's walk through the example we've been using.

For the person who wants to get to 200 lbs.:

- Your protein is set at 200g which equals 800 calories.

- Your fat is set at 65g which equals 585 calories.

- Your total calorie goal is 2400 so you'd subtract 585 and 800 from that number.

- This leaves you with 1,015 calories.

- Divide that number by 4 and you have 255g of carbs (I rounded 253 to 255 to make it easier).

Congrats you've set your starting calorie and macro goals!

This is just the starting point and you'll most likely have to adjust as you go. Every 2-3 weeks be sure to monitor your weight loss. If you're losing more than 2-3 lbs per week — go ahead and increase your calories by 5-10% (in this example you'd up calories by 240) by increasing carbs, fats or both — your preference. Leave protein untouched for the most part (unless you throw in a lower protein day or phase — which we will touch on shortly.) If you're not seeing changes in the mirror, losing inches or seeing the scale trending down after 2-3 weeks I'd lower calories by 5-10% and take away carbs, fats or both depending on your food preference.

MUSCLE GAIN

The only difference between fat loss and muscle gaining goals is the number of calories you'll aim for. If you're looking to gain muscle, simply take your current bodyweight and multiply it by 14. For example, if you currently weigh 200 lbs. you'd aim for 2800 calories. Keep protein the same as the suggestions for fat loss and simply add carbs, fats or both to accommodate your higher calorie goals.

You might be thinking "this seems too simple," and I agree! The fitness industry loves to complicate things to make it seem impossible to find the right formula for achieving your goals, but in reality, things don't have to be that hard. You simply need to start with an educated guess and then adjust based off how your body responds.

The real key is being super consistent so that you can get a clear understanding of how your body is responding to certain calories and macros.

TREAT MEALS NOT CHEAT MEALS

Cheat meals and cheat days somehow have become a "standard" when trying to get in shape. This involves eating as much as you want for a single meal or a whole day every week. This "cheat" strategy started due to highly restrictive diets — especially the bodybuilder style diet — that only allowed for a handful of different foods and required unnecessary levels of dedication to stick to. Unfortunately, this whole cheating thing doesn't work the way people think it does.

Cheat days are just flat out one of the worst strategies you can implement. Gorging and binge eating for a full day is not only unhealthy but is a sure-fire way to completely sabotage your progress. If you're feeling the urge or desire to eat till you feel sick, something needs to change in your plan.

Instead of "cheating" on your diet — which sounds horrible to begin with — my suggestion is to incorporate ways of treating yourself. A treat meal might be a meal that fits your calories but contains somewhat unhealthy food that you're craving. An example might be ice cream or a couple slices of greasy pizza. An occasional treat meal can go a long way in keeping you mentally in the game. Personally, I incorporate 1 or 2 treat meals that fit my calorie goals each week.

As far as full days of eating more calories go — occasionally it makes perfect sense to increase calories for a day or even two. This doesn't mean that you should binge eat or stuff yourself to the point of feeling nauseous. Instead, a controlled increase in calories makes a lot more sense to ensure you aren't setting yourself way back or destroying days of progress.

TRACKING PROGRESS

If you're putting serious effort into your nutrition and workouts - you're going to want to know if you're actually making progress. How do you know if things are working? Should you rely exclusively on the scale? What about progress pictures? Let's outline a simple strategy to see if things are moving in the right direction.

I tell my online clients to follow a detailed, but simple, strategy when it comes to tracking progress. First, never rely on body-fat tracking devices. They are highly inaccurate and will only serve to frustrate you week to week.

When it comes to the scale I have my online clients weigh in first thing in the morning after using the bathroom before they drink or eat anything. They simply record their weight and after 14 days we take the 14-day average. Weight can go up and down based on all kinds of different of factors — therefore, taking a bigger sample size ensures the daily fluctuations aren't clouding your judgement of progress (or lack thereof).

Next, we use measurements. I have my clients measure their chest, arms, waist, hips, and thighs. Taking measurements on the same time of day every 2 weeks makes the most sense for most clients. Measurements combined with weigh-ins can paint a very accurate picture of progress, but we aren't done yet.

Progress pictures (front, side and back) get taken every 4 weeks. It's so hard to see visible changes when you look in the mirror each day, so taking pictures every 4 weeks will help you take note of your physical changes.

Last, each week it's important to get clear on your lifestyle factors. This includes sleep, stress, workout and nutrition adherence. I have my clients rate themselves on a scale of 1-5 (1 being poor and 5 being excellent) on those 4 areas. High levels of negative stress and lack of sleep can bring fat loss to a screeching halt. Plus, if you're only 75% compliant with your workout plan and 60% consistent with your nutrition plan, you'll be able to be very objective when it comes to your progress.

Tracking progress within this framework ensures that you don't overreact to slow progress and that you don't give up before breaking through to new levels of success. Plus, you won't give too much attention to the scale or the mirror. Instead you'll have a well-oiled progress tracking machine that keeps you mentally in the game as you make permanent changes to your body and lifestyle.

06

How to Eat in Any Situation

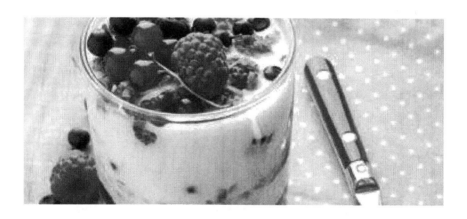

"Getting in shape is like an amusement park. There will be some ups and downs, waiting for results, and lots of food and distractions. Stay active, have fun and, most importantly, enjoy the ride."

Josiah Novak

Life happens and to be honest, life is amazing. Food should never be an unbearable stressor that prevents you from truly enjoying life's precious moments. Birthdays, weddings, nights out with friends, your hometown team in the big game, a big business meeting and numerous other events typically come with food and it's important to have a plan that makes sense so that you can enjoy yourself and, more importantly, be present in the moment to create memories that will last forever. Food can be enjoyed, and you can still make progress.

In this section we're going to outline specific strategies for common situations that you might find yourself in throughout the course of your life so that, if you choose, you'll always have a plan.

PARTIES

Birthdays, weddings, and any big celebrations fall into the categories of parties. I've yet to attend a party that doesn't include either food, alcohol or both. Usually it's a combination. I've been to some epic parties that have an unreal amount of food and I've also been to parties where it's just alcohol and appetizers. Either way, there's calories involved when you attend a party.

Let's get something super clear up front. You have a choice here. You could opt for the "screw it, it's only one night" choice. I won't judge you, and you shouldn't beat yourself up if you decide to go in this direction. This would involve eating and drinking without any clear strategy.

My only warning here is that — depending on where you are in your journey to a healthier version of you — this may temporarily crush your momentum. I might be able to get away with a night of doing whatever I feel like doing simply because I've built good habits over the past decade or so. You might be 10 days into a journey towards the body and lifestyle you want, therefore it wouldn't make sense to go completely off the rails. It might take 10 days for you to get back on track versus a day for someone else who's been living a healthy lifestyle for quite some time.

My point here is that you always have a choice. A plan is worthless without action. If you want to enjoy yourself, and still stay on track, the strategies for parties (and all situations) work very well. However, you might be the type of person that feels overwhelmed and stressed out by having to plan for social events. Do your best. Live your life but understand that results might come slower if you choose the "screw it" route.

For optimal results and to avoid completely going off the rails at parties of any kind is to first game plan for the daytime prior to the party (assuming the party is in the evening). My suggestion is to focus on eating lean low-fat protein sources (chicken, tuna, Greek yogurt, egg whites, etc.) along with green veggies during the day. Assuming you eat 2 times prior to the party, you'll go to the event with quite a few calories left to play with plus most of those calories will be fats and carbs (which will make up most of the party food).

While at the party I suggest a couple strategies. The first is to only eat one plate of food. You can fill it up to your heart's content but stick to one plate. As far as dessert goes, have 1 slice of cake or 2 small treats. If you're drinking alcohol, I have a strategy called 1-2-1-2. It goes like this: have 1 drink then 2 glasses or bottles of water, then repeat.

If these strategies feel way too strict, here's my suggestion. First of all, try it. You won't know how you actually feel about them until you give it a try. Next, do the opposite. Go bananas at your next event and then see how you feel the next day. If you feel good and ready to get back to your normal routine — great! If you feel like crap, then it's probably a good idea to give my strategies a shot.

The choice is yours of course. The good news is that you have the final say in what you do — but remember, take ownership for both the choice in strategy and the results that come. Most of all, enjoy yourself — life's too short to not have fun on a regular basis.

BUSINESS MEETINGS AND LUNCHES

Your job is on the line. This sale must happen. Negotiations are heating up. You take a big client out for a lunch meeting and the last thing you want is to look "weird" for skipping the meal or ordering a boring salad with a water. Being a "health freak" can, at times, make others feel uncomfortable. This of course has nothing to do with you, but in turn it's their own insecurity that's making them feel a bit uneasy. However, there's a way to win on both fronts. You can eat out and still stay on track with your weight loss goals and simultaneously make your business associates feel at ease by "blending in" with their standard business lunch.

The first step is doing your best to plan ahead. There's an above average chance that you know where you're going to eat. Take 2 minutes and dig up the menu online. A simple Google search will most likely lead you to the restaurant's menu where you can do some pre-gaming to ensure that you're clear on what to order once the meeting is underway. Pick a meal that will keep you on track but won't put you under the spotlight (unless that's what you want). Personally, I love when people throw jabs for "eating healthy" — but then again, I run a body transformation company.

Next, be sure to check out the calorie breakdown in My Fitness Pal.[1] Now, you could opt for eyeballing it and you may wind up doing that, however it's rather simple to find caloric information that allows you to fill in the meal just as you would eat your normal choices. Obviously, you may eat more calories than normal, but I have a trick to help you avoid that scenario if you so choose.

My third and final suggestion is to order a power salad when eating out for a business meeting. A protein based, high-fiber, and nutrient packed bowl of healthy and delicious foods goes a long way in doing a couple key things. It shows that you care about your health, but without doing the whole, "can you grill my chicken and ensure it doesn't ever touch butter?" Or the whole, "can the cook make my meal without any oils and is the bread here Gluten Free?" Plus, you'll stay focused on the business meeting because a salad is very easy to eat without thinking about things too much. Not to mention you won't get a massive carb overload as you might with a big bowl of pasta or a gigantic rice platter.

Whatever you do, stay focused on the purpose of the meeting and don't get stressed out about a few extra calories. Do your best and use the strategies listed here — you'll be just fine.

CELEBRATIONS AND FAMILY EVENTS

Listen — have a slice of cake. Yes, A SLICE. Not the whole cake. Certain days and events are incredibly special and worrying about calories and macros just isn't something you should invest your energy in. It's ok to indulge here and there. Your kid's birthday or

---

1   https://www.myfitnesspal.com/

a family event should be enjoyed and avoiding a slice of delicious cake might do you more harm than good.

Sure, I could have told you to fill up on protein and stay focused on your goals — which by the way is totally fine if that's what you decide to do. However, I'd be a total hypocrite if I said that you should avoid sweets and the delicious food at these types of events. You might bump into me at a birthday party one day and I'd hate for you to catch me red-handed eating a mouth-watering slice of carrot cake.

The best advice I can give for a scenario such as a monumental family get together, or a meaningful birthday is to enjoy the moments and be present. If you're following a lifestyle-friendly plan and you've been consistent there's no reason that a slice of cake (with a scoop of ice cream) will completely ruin your progress. In fact, if you can't enjoy these days — what can you really enjoy? Eat a slice of cake, enjoy it, and then get back on track the next day.

TRAVELING

The hardest part of traveling has to be finding ways to stay on track with your nutrition program. Sitting in an airport or driving across the country comes with a bombardment of fast food and other high-calorie options.

A great tool that will help you stay on track is the My Fitness Pal app and website.[2] This is a calorie/macronutrient counter that allows you to track literally everything you eat. This tracking will give you the freedom to fit a lot of different foods into your daily plan. This app has

---

2   https://www.myfitnesspal.com/

a HUGE database with pretty much every restaurant's meals included with the macro and calorie breakdown.

So, if you're sitting at the airport looking around for something to eat, pull up the app and start doing some quick research on what options you have! Because My Fitness Pal and other tracking apps have a huge database of foods from basically every major restaurant as well as generic items you can truly track your calories no matter where you eat. This is vital to a successful travel schedule because your options aren't limited to food that you've prepped.

My clients who travel a lot tend to do well with a couple different strategies. One is to simply go "keto" style while traveling. This involves simply eating protein, fats, and green veggies. Once you're back from your trip you'd reintroduce carbs and get back to a balanced plan. The other strategy is to incorporate carb back-loading. This involves sticking to mostly protein with a little bit of fat during the day and then your last meal of the night can have a significant portion of carbs included. These strategies are simply there to help control caloric intake and make your food choices simple and easy.

When we prepare for our travel plans we often neglect to come prepared with snack options and are forced to find things in the airport, train station or resort to kill our cravings. I highly suggest packing some inexpensive and healthy snacks that will help you avoid major cravings and also keep you satisfied till you can eat a larger meal. Here are some of my suggestions:

1. Turkey or Chicken Jerky

Old fashioned beef jerky is packed with fat and often sugar too. I suggest going for chicken or turkey jerky. There are some really tasty options out there for you to choose from. These snacks are packed with protein without the heavy dose of carbs and fats.

2. Protein Bars and Cookies

More companies are getting on board with healthy protein bars. While I don't suggest you get a majority of your calories from these options, I still think they are great for snacks. Some of my favorite brands are Quest Bars, Icon Meals Cookies, and soon Cellucor will have a healthy protein bar too.

3. Rice Cakes and Peanut Butter

This is one of my all-time favorite snacks. And if you have kids they will love these too! Pack a small jar of peanut butter or almond butter along with a small bag of rice cakes. Combine the two and you'll be thanking me later!! Make sure to opt for the flavored rice cakes ... mmmm good!

4. Apple and Almond Butter

This is a delicious snack that is easy to prep and take with you wherever you go! Cut up an apple and spread some delicious almond butter on the slices!

Treat travel time as a chance to get creative with your eating options. Don't stress being perfect. Nail your calories, make the healthiest choices possible and get back to your normal routine once your trip is over.

07
Your Nutrition Toolkit

"Being healthy is unselfish. Choosing to be unhealthy is selfish."

Josiah Novak

INTERMITTENT FASTING

Intermittent Fasting, for the purpose of this book, refers to going longer-than-normal periods of time without consuming any calories. For example, if your first meal is normally at 8am and you decide to wait till 12pm, you've officially done intermittent fasting. Technically we all intermittently fast. When we sleep, unless you're the person who sleep walks to the peanut butter (yes there are people who do this), you aren't eating while you sleep. That'd be not only weird, but pretty dangerous (and messy). Those 6-8 hours without food is a very small fast.

The intermittent fasting movement, started by Martin Berkhan and his Lean Gains Method,[1] has been turned into a "magical fat loss"

---

1   https://amzn.to/2PNXcoy

tool by certain health and fitness personalities. The idea that you didn't have to eat every 2-3 hours or right when you woke up was unheard of prior to Berkhan's ideas around fasting. He proposed that an 8-hour window was the ideal timeframe for eating. He suggested that your first meal start around noon and then your last finish up around 8pm. Berkhan didn't claim any magical fat loss results, but what he did propose was that eating more calories at each meal and less total meals made more sense for busy people with a lot on their plate.

I was one of those people that bought into intermittent fasting right away.

Intermittent fasting is most definitely not for everyone, nor should most people fast every day. Personally, my body (and mind) feels really good when I wait 3-6 hours after I wake up to eat my first meal. I'm simply not hungry nor do I have any desire to eat first thing in the morning. I'm usually the hungriest at night before bed which fits right into the fasting protocol of having larger meals at night. There are occasions where I'll eat a bit earlier, but rarely do I eat during the first few hours of my day.

If you've always eaten an early morning meal, but you're curious about fasting — let me be the first to say it's not a magical fat loss pill. However, it might help you set up a plan that makes more sense for your lifestyle. If you're not that hungry in the morning but have a raging appetite at night — then it might be worth incorporating the occasional fast.

Longer fasts (20-72 hours) should be approved by a doctor before attempting. There are more health benefits when it comes to longer fasts — such as improved gut health, improved digestion and a more manageable appetite. If you're curious to hear more about the health benefits of intermittent fasting I'd suggest checking out the study by Roger Collier, *Intermittent Fasting: The Science of Going Without*.[2]

My standard recommendation for my online coaching clients is to give at least 12 hours between your final meal before bed and your first meal the next day. This tends to work great for most people. Others can occasionally go longer (14-20 hours), but that's on a case by case basis.

FLEXIBLE NUTRITION

Flexible nutrition, or flexible dieting, refers to the idea that you can eat a variety of different foods as long as you're hitting your daily calories and nutrient goals. This goes against the old "eat chicken, rice and broccoli 4-6 times a day" meal plan that was promoted by bodybuilders and other fitness celebrities for years.

Flexible nutrition is a very simple approach. Eating a variety of healthy foods is encouraged as long as you're controlling your calories and nutrient intake. You can also fit in a few "treats" a couple times a week without blowing your diet as long as you're hitting your calorie and nutrient requirements.

By enjoying a variety of quality food plus a few treats here and there, you'll be much more likely to stick to a diet long term and create a lifestyle that can be enjoyed for the rest of your living years. You no longer have to only be healthy for short spurts. Instead you can take life by the balls and enjoy the food this world has to offer while taking care of yourself.

---

2   https://www.ncbi.nlm.nih.gov/pmc/articles/PMC3680567/

For example, you might decide that Friday nights are pizza nights with the family, but you don't want to blow your hard work from the week. Instead of binge eating on pizza, you can save enough calories for 1-3 slices depending on your targets for the day. That way you'll enjoy great food and create even greater memories while not having to refrain from eating some pizza with the family.

I strongly recommend the smartphone app My Fitness Pal to help track foods that you'd like to fit in your daily meal plan. It pays huge dividends to look up foods at restaurants or foods that you haven't eaten before to learn the nutrition content and fit them in your diet.

The only time I suggest caution with flexible nutrition is if you battle with binge eating on certain foods. I'd suggest establishing some really good habits and cautiously enjoying some "trigger" foods but only when absolutely necessary.

My fellow fitness colleague, James Smith, of James Smith Academy, talks about the Intensity Factor when it comes to food.[3] Certain foods trigger an incredibly strong craving and appetite response in certain people. For me anything with peanut butter and chocolate is difficult to eat in moderation. Nutella, Kit-Kats, and peanut butter flavored foods don't last long in my house. Therefore, my intensity factor is super high (10 out of 10 in this case). There're a couple ways of dealing with this. One, you can avoid those foods altogether or, if you decide to consume them, be cautious and try and mentally prepare yourself. The other option is to replace them with similar foods that are more calorically controlled. For example, full-fat ice cream might be a high-intensity food for you. Instead of never eating ice cream

---

3   https://www.jamessmithacademy.com/

you could replace it with Halo Top or another low-calorie ice cream to cut back on the total calories consumed and avoid an all-out binge.

FRUIT SNACKING AND SPARKLING WATER

Transforming your body and mastering a healthy nutrition plan is far from easy. There are those of you reading this who will struggle with cravings and staying on track with your plan from time to time. I'll raise my hand and own up to the fact that there are days that I really struggle too — especially with cravings.

I interviewed a guy, Greg O'Ghallager, on my *True Transformation Podcast*, who runs a company called Kinobody[4] and he shared with me a couple strategies that, after implementing, really helped with cravings and warding off spikes in appetite.

The first was strategic fruit snacking. Munching on an apple or some berries in between meals when you're feeling that strong urge to hit the vending machine for a chocolate bar can be a huge help in staying on point. High fiber, lower calorie fruits like apples, pears, grapefruit and berries can be a great ally in the fight against cravings.

Sparkling water is another great tool to help you stay on track with your nutrition plan. There's something incredibly satiating and refreshing when it comes to sparkling water. If you've ever been a soda drinker, you'll appreciate the refreshing taste of quality sparkling water. My favorite go-to is Gerolsteiner or "Young Gerald" as my friend Carter Good and I call it.

---

4   https://kinobody.com/

VEGAN DAYS

For those of you who eat a significant amount of meat, it makes sense to occasionally have a "vegan day" where you avoid meat completely in order to give your digestive system a break. Plus, you'll give your gut a chance to process other sources of protein — primarily from plant-based sources — that will help keep your incredibly valuable gut health in check.

I've noticed a significant increase in energy coupled with an improvement in digestion by including vegan days in my programming. My suggestion is to build in a "meat-free" day at least once every 30 days.

08
The Power Method

"Never forget that there's someone out there with bigger problems and more stress than you who's chasing their dreams down every day."

Josiah Novak

WHAT IS THE POWER METHOD?

I hate fad diets. This is why I created The Power Method. The Power Method is NOT a fad diet, nor will it ever be one. In fact, any "fad" diet could technically be used hand in hand with the Power Method to make that diet 10x better overnight.

The Power Method gives you clarity around how to structure your eating plan to best fit your lifestyle and the things you do each day. Eating is a big part of our lives, so it makes sense to have a structure that gives you flexibility coupled with a clear-cut plan.

The Power Method also has optional tools that can be utilized if it makes sense for your health and lifestyle. Tools such as fasting, carb cycling, and strategic Vegan days are there to utilize if needed.

Most importantly this method is simple, fun, flexible but also clear enough to ensure you stay on track for life. The Power Method isn't a "diet" by any means. It's simply a framework that will help you create a sustainable lifestyle. A lifestyle that will give you the body, the strength, and the energy that you desire.

POWER MORNINGS

Whether you work during the day or overnight, your morning starts when you wake up after your main block of sleep. The first part of your day is crucial to ensure that you're mentally in the game and on track with your goals. Having a routine for the first few hours of the day will accelerate your results and set you up for incredible success during your workday and evenings.

Essentials:

- **Hydrate Upon Waking**

  Drink 1 liter of water (preferably room temperature, but just get it in). For an added boost you can add squeezed lemon juice and a teaspoon of pink Himalayan sea salt to your water.

- **Protein- and Fat-Focused Mornings**

  Your morning meal (if you choose to eat one) should be focused primarily on protein, fats and added greens. This helps stabilize your energy and appetite. Having large amounts of carbs or sugar in the morning isn't recommended unless you have a big workout planned for mid-day. Eggs with spinach and a side of chicken or turkey sausage is the perfect example of a morning POWER meal.

Morning Tools:

- **Gratitude Journaling**

  Take 5 minutes each morning and write down 3 things you're thankful for. This puts your mind in a state of gratitude, plus it gives you perspective on the amazing parts of your life that are often taken for granted.

- **Goal Setting**

  Each morning, after gratitude journaling, write down a few behaviors that you want to nail that day that will help you get closer to your goals. This could be a daily steps goal or how many fruits and veggies you want to eat that day.

- **Intermittent Fasting**

  Fasting is not a requirement, but it's a tool I use almost daily. Waiting 4-6 hours to eat my first meal does wonders for mental clarity, energy, and focus. Plus, it gives me more calories to play with as I feast later in the day and evening. Fasting is not required, but I suggest trying it at least once to see how you feel. During fasting hours water, coffee with minimal cream, and tea are permitted.

POWER SALADS

For years, my mid-day meal was a problem. I'd eat a meal with little to no nutritional value and super carb heavy. This caused me to feel super sleepy, unmotivated and lazy from 2pm to the evening time. This was highly detrimental to my progress when it came to sticking to a plan. I'd miss workouts and end up battling big cravings most of the afternoon.

I had been against having salads for a long time simply because salads seemed so damn boring. I mean who wants to eat a bowl of lettuce for a meal? Well, that all changed when I discovered power salads.

I was eating at restaurant one day and I ordered a Mexican Tortilla Salad. This salad was massive. Tons of greens, tomatoes, salsa, avocado, tortilla strips, chicken and some light dressing. It was delicious and satisfying. I felt great after eating it and when I looked up the calories I felt even better. For 400-500 calories I got a tasty, nutritious and incredibly energizing meal. Plus, I didn't feel an energy crash afterwards. I wasn't even hungry for the next 6 hours. I started to think that salads might be my mid-day solution. I started trying different combinations of ingredients at home and then when I'd eat out I would order the salad options at different restaurants. Salads quickly became my go-to mid-day tool.

Getting quality nutrients and controlling your energy while satisfying your appetite isn't always easy. However, power salads do all of that in one meal. Having a mid-day meal centered around greens (which provide nutrients, fiber and take up a lot of room in your stomach) along with added nutrients from fruit, lean protein, and healthy fats will help you stay on track and full of clear energy for the remainder of your day.

It's important to remember that calories still count here. Don't bother worrying about tracking the leafy green veggies, but be sure to stay aware of added proteins, nuts, fruits, dressing or other higher calorie additions. I've included my favorite Power Salad combinations in the resources section.

POWER HOUR

Getting 60 minutes of activity each day is crucial for health, life, mindset and happiness. Some days you might fill this time with an organized workout built around weights, mobility and cardio work. Other days you might go on a hike with your friends or maybe go on a nice jog around your city or neighborhood. You might take a 30 minute walk some days and then do a quick 30-minute home workout later in the day. 60 minutes of activity each day is the goal here. This doesn't have to be done all in one shot. You can break it up as you see fit, but get it done and enjoy it. This is how you build energy and endurance for all that life throws at you.

In the bonus resources section — you have workout recommendations for a month ahead. Commit to 60 minutes of movement per day and you will build a strong and healthy foundation for success in all areas of your life.

POWER SMOOTHIE

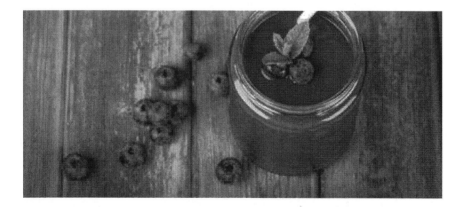

We've been conditioned to eat, snack, eat some more, snack some more and then eat again. This around the clock feeding schedule can lead to your brain getting used to having food every couple of hours which can then lead to appetite swings throughout the day. These hunger signals can't always be trusted. Often times you're simply bored or just following the usual eating routine that you've trained your brain to follow.

Instead of telling you to stop snacking completely (something I do suggest trying to move towards eventually), my recommendation is a Power Smoothie.

The Power Smoothie is another nutrient packed, satisfying, delicious and convenient piece to the Power Method. Smoothies are easy to make and can knock out a sweet tooth pretty fast.

Technically the Power Smoothie could be the first meal you have each day if you're rushing out of the house and don't have time to make a meal. They can also serve as a nice bridge between your Power Salad and Power Feast.

A smoothie might also help tide you over from your first meal to a late lunch. Whichever option you choose, the smoothie is the swiss army knife for nutrition plans.

The Power Smoothie is not required, but I suggest utilizing one consistently if you find that you're reaching for snacks or battling sugar cravings. I've included my favorite Power Smoothie Recipes in the resources section of the book.

POWER FEAST

Last but not least is the Power Feast. The Power Feast is your largest meal of the day. Most people struggle with eating after a long day of work, stress, family obligations, and other life related responsibilities. When you're stressed out and exhausted the last thing on your mind is sticking to a small, calorie-controlled meal that helps you lose body fat. You want a satisfying meal that gives you a full stomach as you wind down for the day. Not to mention your social events tends to revolve around food and eating with loved ones, therefore it makes sense to have your largest meal towards the end of your waking hours.

The Power Feast isn't an excuse to binge nor is it a requirement if you prefer to sleep on a light stomach. For me, and most of my clients, this piece is tremendously helpful when it comes to staying consistent and enjoying life. You'll still want to center this meal around healthy food choices that make you feel great. You can also sneak in some healthier forms of dessert if your calorie goals allow for it — such as Greek yogurt with fruit or some healthier versions of ice cream.

Personally, I save about 40-50% of my daily calories for this last meal. This comes out to about 1200 calories for me that I utilize to have a sizeable dinner along with a healthier dessert. I suggest playing around with this and figuring out what works best for you. You may find that a smaller percentage of your daily calories makes you feel better or you may even go with a higher percentage if you tend to enjoy that more. The most important thing is that you hit your calorie targets based on your goals along with getting sufficient protein. Everyone is different when it comes to what works best for setting up a nutrition plan. Do what works the best and enjoy the process.

You'll find my favorite "feasts" recipes in the resources section on my website.

09

How to Keep the Weight Off

"The real work starts once you've accomplished a big goal. The ability to set new goals and keep challenging yourself is what separates good from great."

Josiah Novak

This world doesn't have a weight loss problem. Just look around and you'll see thousands of before and after pictures around the internet. People are losing weight every day. The real issue is that people can't seem to keep the weight off. You drop 20 lbs. only to see it slowly pile back on.

There're quite a few factors behind this phenomenon of weight loss followed by weight gain. First, is appetite. Studies have shown that people who lose a lot of weight have higher than normal appetites following a weight loss phase.[1] This is mostly due to your body

---

1   https://www.webmd.com/diet/news/20161014/how-your-appetite-can-
     sabotage-weight-loss#2

having a set point for your weight. The body doesn't want to drop below it's set point so your appetite increases. This is primarily due to a hormone called Leptin, who's main function in the body is long-term appetite control. When there's enough fuel in the body from body-fat Leptin levels go up which signal the brain to stop eating. However, over the course of a fat loss phase, leptin levels steadily trend down which increases appetite and leads to over-eating. It's no wonder that people's will-power runs out. They're literally fighting their body to maintain their weight loss.

There've also been studies showing that those who are obese have what's known as Leptin Resistance.[2] This is when the leptin is being created by the body, but the signal isn't being recognized in the brain. This causes huge issues for people who are already overweight but just can't seem to control their appetite. They keep eating and eating and the weight continues to pile on.

The other hunger hormone known as Ghrelin, which is secreted by the stomach, is a short-term appetite regulator. Its primary role is to signal your body to eat when the stomach is empty.

Ghrelin is highest before a meal and lowest afterwards. When it comes to losing weight, controlling Ghrelin is crucial. Eating higher protein meals, avoiding crash diets, and getting enough sleep are crucial to controlling appetite — especially ghrelin.[3]

Long term weight loss maintenance also revolves around your mental approach to this whole fitness journey. Most people treat getting in shape as a race to the finish. They think about their goals as an end-date. What if we reversed this? What if achieving your

2   https://www.precisionnutrition.com/leptin-ghrelin-weight-loss
3   https://draxe.com/ghrelin/

goal was simply the starting point? Losing those 20 lbs. becomes the foundation for a lifelong pursuit of health and fitness instead of a temporary phase.

It's time to quit looking at getting in shape as a temporary project. Fitness and health need to become the foundation that you build your entire routine around. Staying active, eating healthy and taking care of your body can't be done for just 90 days. It's great to look at the before and after pictures and think that once you get in shape the work is done. However, the work is just starting.

Bruce Lee famously said, "Don't pray for an easy life. Pray for the strength to endure a difficult one." I truly believe that the work begins once you've arrived at your ideal level of health and fitness. The work it took to get there still needs to be done. This is why my online clients get put on a maintenance phase at regular intervals to protect their weight loss. It's not enough to drop pounds and then think that the weight will stay off just because you did the work to get there.

In my experience, it takes about 6-12 months for your body to adapt to the weight loss and create a new "set point" where it's comfortable being at a lower weight. Everyone is different when it comes to this adaptation, but I've noticed that clients who work really hard to maintain their weight loss efforts seem to gradually notice the body getting more comfortable around the 6-12 month mark. This doesn't mean they can go back to eating whatever they want and avoiding activity. However, hunger seems to be more controllable and appetite is a bit easier to regulate around that timeframe.

You'll need to test things out for yourself of course but be prepared to maintain your weight loss with the same focus and discipline that helped you lose the weight in the first place.

Gradually increasing calories (200-300 per week) after a calorie restriction phase is a great way to begin the maintenance phase. If you see your weight and body start to gain weight, be patient and stay at your calorie level until things begin to level out.

This "reverse diet" strategy is not easy. Adding calories back in can spike appetite and the body will begin to really crave more food. If you go into this reverse phase expecting this jump in hunger, you'll be prepared to battle with your body's hormonal reaction. This won't be easy, but it's a necessary undertaking if you're going to avoid the dreaded rebound and weight gain standard that has been set.

HABITS, ROUTINES AND ENVIRONMENT

Staying fit and healthy will always come down to the habits and routines that you practice each day. The habit experts talk about it taking 60+ days to build habits that last, but my thought is that habits require consistent attention. In order to continue down the path of health and fitness — you must consistently build your life around the habits, routines and rituals that give you the desired outcomes you desire.

Combining healthy habits with a strong and supportive environment is crucial for maintaining your results (as well as continuing to improve). If you're surrounded by people who don't support your goals or who aren't living a healthy lifestyle, it will be challenging to stay on top of your health and fitness routine.

I can't emphasis enough the importance of setting up your environment for success. Get rid of the unhealthy food that you have no chance of avoiding in your house, separate yourself from negative influences and avoid distractions that only serve to pull you away from your goals.

Living a life on your terms that is fulfilling, long-lasting and full of abundance comes down to the habits you choose to enforce and the environment you decide to live in.

10
Companies You Should Follow

"If you're the smartest, most talented and most successful person in the room — you're in the wrong room. Always surround yourself with people who push you to improve in all areas of life."

Josiah Novak

The fitness industry is jam packed with people trying to sell you stuff. Pills, powders, and programs are everywhere. Of course, I'm biased, but I truly think this book is the best nutrition book on the planet and if you follow the program I've laid out here, this will be the only book on nutrition you'll ever need.

However, I'm humble enough to know that I'm not the smartest nor am I the only person you should connect with in the industry. My online coaching program transforms thousands of lives each year, but there are other amazing people and companies doing incredible things in the industry. his chapter is all about putting a spotlight on the people who have, dare I say, changed my life and helped True

Transformation become the incredible organization that it is and continues to be each day.

JASON PHILLIPS – IN3 NUTRITION

https://in3nutrition.com/

Jason is not only one of the smartest people on the planet when it comes to nutrition, he also happens to be one of my best friends in the industry. His business is centered around making an impact in people's lives and he continues to set the standard for what over-delivering looks like. Be sure to follow him and his brand IN3 Nutrition.

MIND PUMP MEDIA – ADAM, SAL, JUSTIN AND DOUG

https://www.mindpumpmedia.com/

Mind Pump burst onto the scene around the same time that I started True Transformation. The Mind Pump Podcast is my #1 podcast that I not only listen to but refer to other people as well. The guys at Mind Pump are a must-follow if you're looking to learn about health and fitness. I predict that Mind Pump will become a household name in the next 5 years or less. I'm proud to call these guys friends — be sure to follow them and listen to their podcast — I was a guest on episode 692.

JEREMY SCOTT

https://www.jeremyscottfitness.com/

If you're looking for a no-BS approach to training, living life and working your ass off — Jeremy Scott is the man. His Instagram, podcast and Blogs are incredibly valuable. His work ethic is always pushing me to take my effort to new levels.

THE ONLINE COACH – RAYMOND QUERIDO

https://the-online-coach.com/

Raymond is a fellow Dad (to 3 kids!) and his consistency with putting out quality and helpful content is second to none. His YouTube channel has helped thousands of people (including me) and he's always sharing his life as a father, husband, entrepreneur and all-around good dude. He's helped me with my nutrition plan and I encourage you to check him out!

GHOST LIFESTYLE – RYAN AND DAN

https://www.ghostlifestyle.com/

Dan Lourenco and Ryan Hughes are making waves in the supplement industry. Their GHOST supplement and lifestyle company are leading a movement backed by truth and science when it comes to using supplementation properly. They have quickly built a team of hard-working, intelligent and charismatic athletes who are all great examples of how to balance fitness with life.

CHASE CHEWNING – EVER FORWARD RADIO

https://chasechewning.com/

Chase Chewning's Ever Forward brand is centered around expanding your life and pushing forward through life's challenges. Chase is a phenomenal coach as well as a leading example of how to utilize fitness to improve all areas of life.

RYAN MICHLER – ORDER OF MAN

https://www.orderofman.com/

Ryan is not a "fitness" guy, but his movement, Order of Man, is one that you should pay attention to. If you're looking for clarity around how to improve your life and become a person of value — Ryan is your guy. Ryan and I both agree that getting your health and fitness in order is the first place to start when working on improving your life. I appeared on Order of Man Podcast on episode 148.

CARTER GOOD

https://www.cartergood.com/

Carter's transformation is inspiring, and he continues to provide massive value to his audience. He's one of the best resources when it comes to learning how to balance having a fun lifestyle while still getting in incredible shape. Carter is also a great friend and we co-host The Moscow Mule Podcast.

AMANDA BUCCI

https://www.amandabucci.com/

Amanda Bucci is one of the most transparent and hardworking entrepreneurs in the health, fitness and lifestyle space. Amanda gained a massive following by sharing her ups and downs with her own fitness journey. In a world full of people only sharing highlight reels, Amanda was one of the first to get real and share the good, bad and the ugly. She now helps up and coming entrepreneurs find their authentic voice to help share their message with the world.

JAMIE ALDERTON

https://www.grenade-fit.com/

Jamie was one of the first business mentors I ever had. Besides being one of the fittest men on earth, Jamie is also one of the kindest people I've ever met. Jamie took my fitness business from barely making any money to giving me the blueprint that allowed me to touch thousands of lives. I can't thank Jamie enough for his guidance and if you're someone who needs help with life, fitness or business — Jamie is your man.

MARTIN BERKHAN

https://leangains.com/

Despite the fact that I don't agree with the recent methods that he released in his book (specifically his extremely high protein recommendation) — The Lean Gains Method — I have to give Martin tremendous props for his work around intermittent fasting. Martin's No-BS style and commitment to research inspired me to try things outside of the norm. Martin is a class act and supplies his following with a wealth of information.

MIKE VACANTI

http://www.ontheregimen.com/

Mike is one of the best online and in-person fitness trainers I've had the chance to meet in the industry. He also created an easy to use Macro Tracking app called Mike's Macros — which some of my clients use to track their food intake.

JORDAN SYATT

https://www.syattfitness.com/

If there was an award for the nicest guy in Fitness — I think Jordan would win hands down. I've become friends with Jordan and I've invested into learning from him and I must say — this guy is the real deal. His work ethic and commitment to his tribe is tremendously inspiring.

EMILY HAYDEN

https://www.thetruetransformation.com/podcast/111-how-to-evolve-with-emily-hayden/

Emily's story is very similar to mine. Coming from an abusive household, being homeless and suffering from depression — Emily's road in life has been far from easy. Emily now leads hundreds of thousands of people on a movement based around Evolving as a person. Her message resonates with me and I highly suggest you give her a follow.

TONY STEPHAN

https://tonystephandietitian.com/

Tony Stephan is one of the best online nutrition coaches in the game. His passion for helping others and his consistent positive energy will inspire you as well as educate you. He's also a tremendous business coach if you're an up and coming online entrepreneur.

CODY "BOOM BOOM" MCBROOM

https://boomboomperformance.com/

Cody is the only guy I've met in fitness who makes me question my own work ethic. This guy puts out so much helpful content. He's an excellent trainer, coach and fellow professional who's driven to help millions. Give him a follow.

JAMES SMITH

https://www.jamessmithacademy.com/

James Smith's edgy, real and hilarious approach to fitness took the U.K. by storm over. His hilarious and often sarcastic approach to health and fitness is a breath of fresh air in the industry riddled with fakes and phonies. James knows his stuff and his content is incredibly straight forward and helpful.

MIKE MATTHEWS

https://www.muscleforlife.com/

Mike is hands down the best writer and content creator I've met in the fitness space. This guy might be the "genius" of the health and fitness industry. Mike is also one of the most humble and down to earth people you'll ever meet. His *Muscle For Life* books and Legion Supplements are of the highest quality.

LARRY HAGNER

https://gooddadproject.com/

Larry's The Good Dad Project podcast focuses on helping Fathers become the best parent, husband, and person they can be. Larry is not only an incredible human being, but a huge proponent of health, fitness and an enjoyable lifestyle. I highly suggest connecting with Larry, especially if you're a father or a soon-to-be Dad.

11
Online Resources

🏆 **Coaching:**
TheTrueTransformation.com/coaching-application

🎙 **Podcast:**
The True Transformation Podcast

f **Facebook Page:**
Facebook.com/JosiahFitness

f **FREE Facebook Group:**
Facebook.com/groups/TrueFitGroup

📷 **Instagram:**
@JosiahFitness

🐦 **Twitter:**
@JosiahFitness

▶ **YouTube:**
YouTube.com/TrueTransform

📂 **For an entire database of resources please visit:**
TheTrueTransformation.com/DietsSuck

ABOUT THE AUTHOR

Josiah Novak is a fitness coach, author, host of the True Transformation Podcast and creator of The True Transformation Body Transformation System.

His lifestyle friendly, real life, simple and long-term focused approach has helped thousands of men and women to achieve permanent results when it comes to their body, fitness, life and health goals. His work has been featured in Fitness RX magazine, Mind Pump Media, Order of Man, and many popular outlets.

He lives in Northern Virginia with his wife Michelle and their two boys, Jaxson and Cameron.

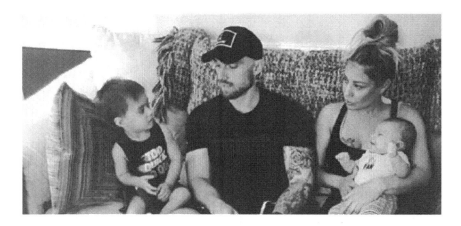

BONUS – TRUE TRANSFORMATION BLUEPRINTS

THE TOP 8 TRANSFORMATION NUTRITION AND WORKOUT PLANS FROM THOUSANDS OF CASE STUDIES

INTRODUCTION

After 15 years of working as a personal trainer and online health and fitness coach, I've had the opportunity to work with and impact thousands of lives. I've put together hundreds of transformation plans and have had tremendous amounts of success working with clients from different walks of life. It would be impossible to put together a resource with every single successful case study I've been a part of. However, after going through my client files, I decided to outline 5 detailed plans that have helped 5 of my best clients over the past decade and a half. All of these clients worked with me virtually thanks to the power of the Internet and each one was highly successful, plus they've kept their results after finishing my program. You'll see that all their backgrounds were different and that each one took a different path when it came to reaching their goals – which illustrates that there isn't a one-size-fits-all approach when it comes to health and fitness.

As you read through this guide — keep in mind that parts of these plans may work for you and parts may not. Getting in shape is highly individual and your plan should be completely customized based around your lifestyle and unique needs. To apply for coaching please visit: TheTrueTransformation.com/Coaching-Application.

CASE STUDIES #1 AND #2: JOSH AND SARAH MARTIN

Background: Josh and Sarah joined my 8 Week Transformation Coaching Program based off a recommendation from another client, Tony, who's featured in this guide. Both wanted to lose body fat, improve their energy and look better in a bathing suit. After having kids, they had let their fitness routine go to the wayside. Life had become a little crazy, but they had come to the realization that they weren't happy with how they looked or felt and they wanted to set a better example for their kids when it came to health and fitness.

The Set-Up

Both Josh and Sarah work full time plus they had numerous family activities on the weekend. Not to mention neither one of them wanted to follow anything too restrictive that prevented them from having a social life and an enjoyable time with their kids. Plus, they couldn't be in the gym for more than 45 minutes a day, 5 times a week due to family obligations. This meant that a heavy emphasis needed to be placed on weight training along with activity outside the gym. Their nutrition plan couldn't be too complicated either. They needed to be able to eat foods their kids like while also have a simple routine to follow during the day. Both enjoy carbohydrates more than heavy amounts of fats, so we kept that in mind. Neither one had religiously tracked their food before, so that needed to be taken into consideration as well. Mentally they were initially skeptical of my methods, which wasn't surprising. The fitness industry is full of scammers, so I was very patient with them and worked hard to build their trust. Both Josh and Sarah, right off the bat, were hard working. In fact, I had to be sure to remind them that this was a long-term process and that they could burn out if they dropped weight and fat too fast.

Josh's Plan

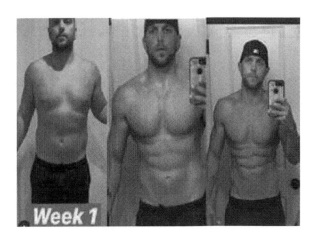

Josh had no problem committing to the gym and was eager to learn how to track his calories. Initially we did a 4-day workout split that had him in the gym 4 times per week. His workout split looked like this:

Day 1: Upper Body

Day 2: Lower Body and Core

Day 3: Off

Day 4: Upper Body

Day 5: Lower Body and Core

Weekends: Optional Workout but Priority on Recovery

Josh's body-fat, in my estimation, was around 23-24% at the start so we kept his nutrition plan very balanced. Typically, the leaner people are the more efficient they are at utilizing carbs in their diet. However, people carrying more bodyfat (for males this is usually over 20%) I tend to keep fats and carbs balanced. This isn't always the rule, but this is the protocol more often than not. At times, if the person is a good fit, we go higher fats to keep their appetite under control and to help them stay consistent at first before we go back to more of a balanced approach. Right from the start Josh was very consistent with his calorie and macro tracking so we kept things balanced as he leaned down.

Once Josh was around 18% bodyfat we started increasing the overall percentage of calories dedicated to carbohydrates. This boosted his performance in the gym tremendously and he had no issue staying consistent. We kept calories as high as possible while monitoring his fat loss very closely. Josh checked in each week and fortunately he stayed very consistent with his dedication and commitment to the plan.

Once Josh was around 15% bodyfat we started incorporating higher calorie days to help him stay mentally on track. Since we never went too extreme with his calorie level, Josh never felt deprived or super hungry. Having a higher calorie day once every 2 weeks or so gave him just enough of a boost to stay on track.

After working with me for about 5 months Josh was very lean. His bodyfat was hovering around 10% which is extremely lean for most guys. He had visible abs and was very happy with how he looked. At this point we decided to push one last time for a beach trip that he and Sarah were both excited about. Josh wanted to show up and look his all-time best. For about 8 weeks we pushed the diet and training to dip to around 7-8% bodyfat. Josh, despite being hungry and a little tired, pushed through like a champion and showed up to the beach looking incredible.

From there, we started his reverse diet. Josh got down to around 200g of carbs a day at his lowest (which is still high for most people who want to get super lean). Josh wanted to stay lean but knew he couldn't eat low calories forever, so we slowly started adding both carbs and fats back to his diet. Over the course of about 6-8 weeks we went from eating 200g of carbs and 50g of fats per day to eating 400g of carbs and 100g of fats per day while maintaining a perfect 6 pack and an enjoyable lifestyle.

Josh is easily one of the most dedicated clients I've ever had. His secret to success? He stayed accountable to me each day with a simple check in via email. We chatted on the phone a few times to ensure he had everything he needed, and he always took my advice and applied it right away. Josh, despite being skeptical at first, completely trusted the process and took massive action each day.

Sample Workout Plan for Josh

Workout 1 (Gym) – Upper Push Workout

Warm Up: 5-10 minutes of treadmill or bike and lightweight for first exercise

Rest: 60 seconds MAX between sets

1) Deadlifts – 3 sets of 10

2) Dips – 4 sets of 6

3) Incline Dumbbell Press – 4 sets of 4

4) Close Grip Bench Press – 5 sets of 5

Can't make it to the gym? – Do this workout:

1) Push-Ups – 12 sets of 10 – but hold the bottom position for a 5 count and the top position for a 5 count.

2) Crab Walks – 20 one way – 20 the other way (5 sets)

Workout 2 (Gym) – Pull Workout

Warm Up: 5-10 minutes of treadmill or bike and lightweight for first exercise

Rest: 90 seconds MAX between sets

1) Barbell Rows – 6 sets 5

2) Deadlifts – 5 sets of 5

3) Rear Delt Dumbbell Flys – 4 sets of 6

4) Barbell Curls – 5 sets of 5

5) Wide Grip Pull-Downs – 4 sets of 6

Can't make it to the gym? – Do this workout:

1) Burpees – 20 seconds on – rest for 10 seconds – repeat for 10 rounds

2) Planks – 30 seconds on – rest for 15 seconds – repeat for 10 rounds

Workout 3 (Gym) – Lower Body

Warm Up: 5-10 minutes of treadmill or bike and lightweight for first exercise

Rest: 90 seconds MAX between sets

1) Squats – 6 sets of 5

2) Standing Calf Raises – 5 sets of 8

3) Leg Press – 5 sets of 5

4) Lying Leg Curls – 5 sets of 5

5) Seated Calf Raises – 5 sets of 8

Can't make it to the gym? – Do this workout:

1) 8 rounds of:
   - 10 Squat Jumps
   - 10 Mountain Climbers
   - 10 Jump Lunges
   - 10 Push-Ups
   - Rest 30 seconds

Cardio: 3 35-minute walks outside or on the treadmill at an average pace

Sarah's Plan

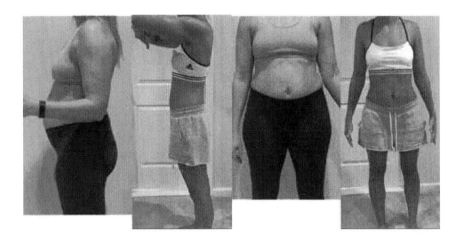

Sarah was new to weight training, so I wanted to ease her into a routine. My requirement initially was 2-3 weight training workouts per week combined with tracking her steps each day. I knew if she could stay active and incorporate resistance training she'd start to see massive returns very quickly. Sarah wanted to drop some stubborn body-fat that she'd added after having kids and she wanted to feel incredible in a bathing suit again. She also needed a plan that was very "Mom Life" friendly. Low carb and low fat were out of the question. She needed to be on a similar plan as Josh to ensure their home life was super enjoyable and convenient.

Sarah's Nutrition Plan

Sarah focused on eating a very balanced meal plan. She kept a high amount of variety simply because of family and date nights being a part of her life on a regular basis. Josh and Sarah both were eating close to the same types of food so that was a huge bonus.

Sample Meal Plan:

- Meal 1: Eggs and Toast

- Meal 2: Protein Smoothie

- Meal 3: Large Green Salad with Fruit and Chicken

- Meal 4: Rice, Fish, and Veggies

Sarah's Starting Workout Plan

Workout 1 (Gym) – Upper Push Workout

Warm Up: 5-10 minutes of treadmill or bike and lightweight for first exercise

Rest: 90 seconds MAX between sets

1) Flat Dumbbell Bench Press – 3 sets of 6-8

2) Seated Dumbbell Shoulder Press – 3 sets of 6-8

3) Tricep Dips – 3 sets of 6-8

4) Machine Chest Press – 3 sets of 6

5) Dumbbell Kickbacks – 3 sets of 6 each arm

Can't make it to the gym? – Do this workout:

1) Push-Ups – 10 sets of 10 – but hold the bottom position for a 5 count and the top position for a 5 count

2) Crab Walks – 20 one way – 20 the other way

Workout 2 (Gym) – Pull Workout

Warm Up: 5-10 minutes of treadmill or bike and lightweight for first exercise

Rest: 90 seconds MAX between sets

1) Barbell Rows – 3 sets 6-8

2) Sumo Deadlifts – 3 sets of 6

3) Rear Delt Dumbbell Flys – 3 sets of 6

4) Barbell Curls – 3 sets of 6-8

5) Wide Grip Pull-Downs – 3 sets of 6-8

Can't make it to the gym? – Do this workout:

1) Burpees – 20 seconds on – rest for 10 seconds – repeat for 8 rounds

2) Planks – 30 seconds on – rest for 15 seconds – repeat for 8 rounds

Workout 3 (Gym) – Lower Body

Warm Up: 5-10 minutes of treadmill or bike and lightweight for first exercise

Rest: 90 seconds MAX between sets

1) Squats – 3 sets of 6-8

2) Dumbbell Walking Lunges – 3 sets of 8 each leg

3) Leg Press – 3 sets of 10

4) Lying Leg Curls – 3 sets of 8

5) Seated Calf Raises – 3 sets of 8

Can't make it to the gym? – Do this workout:

1) 7 rounds of :
    - 10 Squat Jumps
    - 10 Mountain Climbers
    - 10 Jump Lunges
    - 10 Push-Ups
    - Rest 30 seconds

CASE STUDY #3: CHRISTIAN OLANOWSKI

Christian is a younger guy (early twenties) and a former wrestler. Going to college and getting into the daily "adult" life brought on some bad habits that Christian wanted help correcting. He'd looked in the mirror and saw a guy even he didn't recognize. Christian came to me looking to adopt a much healthier lifestyle and get workouts that pushed him out of his comfort zone.

Christian wrote me an email outlining his diet set up (I had him do this so that I could be sure that he was learning the things I teach). Here's what he wrote after working with me for a few months:

"I typically do not follow a very strict "diet," but my eating habits are relatively consistent.

To start my day, I have 1-2 cups of coffee with creme.

Around 10-11am I eat 2 granola/protein bars.

Most of the time I skip lunch, but since I am in outside sales, I typically eat out. I try to go for something as low calorie as possible.

Dinner is relatively consistent recently. I will do 1/2 cup rice, 1 cup of mixed greens, 2 cups of chicken, 1/4-1/2 avocado.

I always have something small at night. Whether it is granola/protein bar or some chicken, it varies."

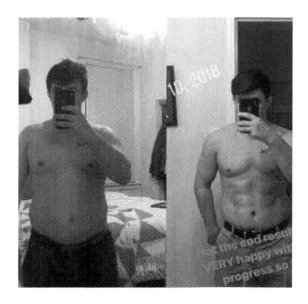

Christian's Starting Workout Plan

Workout 1 – Upper Body

Rest Between Sets: 90 seconds

Active Warm-Up: Push-Ups x 10

1) Flat Dumbbell Bench Press – 3 sets of 8

2) Standing Dumbbell Shoulder Press
   - Week 1-2: 3 sets of 6
   - Week 3-4: 4 sets of 5

3) Dumbbell Row – 3 sets of 10

4) Tricep Rope Push-Downs – 3 sets of 10

5) Cable Bicep Curls – 3 sets of 10

6) Wide Grip Lat Pull-Downs – 2 sets of 10

7) Rope Face-Pulls – 2 sets of 10

Workout 2 – Lower Body

Active Warm-Up: Kettlebell Swings – 2 sets of 8

1) Goblet Squats
   - Week 1-2: 3 sets of 6
   - Week 3-4: 4 sets of 5

2) Leg Press – 3 sets of 10

3) Seated Calf Raises – 3 sets of 10

4) Dumbbell Stiff Leg Deadlifts – 3 sets of 10

5) Planks – 3 reps of 30 seconds

6) Crunches – 3 sets of 20

Workout 3 – Upper Body

Active Warm-Up: Push-Ups – 2 sets of 10

1) Pull-Ups
   - Week 1-2: 3 sets of 6
   - Week 3-4: 4 sets of 5

2) Incline Dumbbell Press – 3 sets of 10

3) Seated Cable Rows – 3 sets of 10

4) Standing Side Laterals with Dumbbells – 3 sets of 10

5) Dumbbell Curls – 3 sets of 10

6) Tricep Dips – 3 sets of 10

Workout 4 – Lower Body

Active Warm-Up: Broad Jumps x 6

1) Pause Squat (pause at bottom)
   - Week 1-2: 3 sets of 5
   - Week 3-4: 4 sets of 3

2) Barbell Reverse Lunges – 3 sets of 8 per leg

3) Standing Calf Raises – 3 sets of 10

4) Back Extensions – 3 sets of 10

5) Bicycle Crunches – 3 sets of 10 per side

CASE STUDY #4: JAMAL SMITH

Jamal came to me looking to improve how he looked with his shirt off, boost his energy and create a lifestyle friendly plan. Jamal is a father, busy professional and enjoys social events with friends and family. Jamal wanted abs but also knew that his family and friends are his biggest priority, so we couldn't sacrifice his social health just for a six pack.

Being a father myself I knew that the plan I created for Jamal needed to factor in meals with his kids and his girlfriend. Jamal wanted the ultimate flexibility with his nutrition plan but also the peace of mind knowing he was on track to meet his fat loss goals. He was 100% committed to tracking his macros so that's the route we went to start.

Here's my first email to him that includes his starting plan:

Jamal Smith Body Transformation Plan

Please read through the following very carefully before reviewing your plan:

- All check ins are due Friday morning by 11:00 am EST. The latest I can accept a weekly check in is 12:30 pm EST on Friday. This is due to me allocating time to deal with client plans and quickly turning around any tweaks or changes you may need. Failure to check in on time will result in having to wait till the following week to make changes.

- Please use the mobile app to input your weight and progress pictures each week.

- We will be having a Skype call once per month to discuss your progress. Please utilize the Voxer app to stay in touch with me via walkie talkie throughout the week as well.

- Timing of your meals is up to you. What's most important is hitting your total protein, carbs and fats each day.

- Make sure you are consuming a minimum of 3-4 liters of water each day on this plan.

- Tweaks and changes to your plan are only made if things aren't progressing. "If it ain't broke don't fix it."

- Workouts and diet are just two pieces to the plan. The third piece is Mindset. A positive mindset is crucial to success whenever trying to obtain new levels of success. Wake up each day and remind yourself why you're doing this!

Nutrition Strategy and Routine

Morning Routine:

1) Weigh Yourself first thing upon waking after using the restroom — record that weight on your notes in your phone and then send me all 7 weigh-ins every Friday.

2) Drink a Liter of Water after weighing yourself.

3) 3x per week squeeze a lemon into your water in the morning

4) 3x per week I want you skipping breakfast (unless you're very hungry) — push your first meal to 3-5 hours after waking up. During this fasting period, you can drink water, green tea or black coffee.

5) On days that you don't fast I want your first meal to be protein and fats only. Something like 2-3 eggs with turkey bacon or avocado.

6) On Fasting days, I suggest breaking your fast with a high protein, moderate carb, low fat meal — for example: Chicken and potatoes or egg whites and oatmeal.

Starting Calories and Macros

The most important thing to remember is that the key to long term success is tracking your food to start to truly learn how much you need to be eating to get lean and stay lean while building muscle.

Please download the My Fitness Pal App on your smartphone — however do NOT follow the guidelines in the app — you can customize your intake goal for the day — use the numbers below

Protein: 180g per day Carbs: 250g per day Fats: 60g per day

Sample Meal Plan (Fasting Days):

- Meal 1: (10-11 am): egg whites Fruit Oatmeal mixed with almond milk

- Meal 2 (2-3 pm): Whey protein shake Peanut Butter

- Meal 3 (6-7 pm): Grilled Chicken with veggies or green salad and Rice

- Meal 5 (before bed): Greek Yogurt and a Protein Bar

Sample Meal Plan (Non-Fasting Days):

- Meal 1: Eggs, Bacon, Avocado

- Meal 2: Whey Protein Shake Rice Cakes

- Meal 3: Turkey or Shrimp Green Veggies Potatoes

- Meal 4: Homemade healthy pizza with turkey pepperoni and ground beef, peppers and onions

Nutrition Strategies

1) One Day Per Week go out for a nice dinner or have 1 meal of anything you're craving. The only rule is that you stop eating once you're full. We will cover this in detail on our first skype call.

2) Eat fish (salmon, cod, or shrimp) at least 2-3x per week.

3) Eat red meat at least 2x per week to optimize testosterone.

4) 2 servings of green veggies per day

5) 1 serving of fruit at least every other day

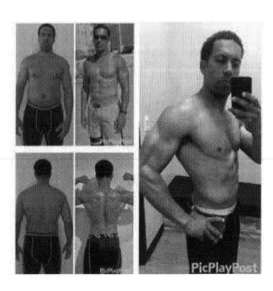

Jamal's Workout Strategy

With workouts I knew Jamal wanted some athletic components along with the "aesthetic" results, so we combined some basic muscle-building routines with some higher intensity athletic style training. I also had Jamal stay active on days he was out of the gym to ensure he was burning a ton of calories.

Here's a breakdown of how Jamal's workout routine was set up:

Day 1 – Chest, Shoulders, Triceps and Abs

Bike or Walk on Treadmill for 5 minutes to break a small sweat

Warm Up: Here is a video that I want you to watch and use to warm up each day

1) Flat Barbell Bench Press – 2 warm up sets – 3 sets of 68

2) Seated Dumbbell Shoulder Press – 2 warm up sets – 3 sets of 68

3) Incline Dumbbell Press – 3 sets of 68

4) Standing Side Laterals with Dumbbells – 3 sets of 8

5) Parallel Bar Dips (add weight if necessary) – 2 sets of 68

6) Rope Push-Downs – 3 sets of 68

7) Rope Crunches – 3 sets of 1215

Cardio Workout (can be performed in the morning or evening): 30 minutes steady pace on step mill, treadmill or elliptical

Day 2 – Back, Biceps and Rear Delts

Walk and Warm Up (same as Day 1)

1) Close Grip Pull-Ups – 4 sets of 68 (add weight if necessary)

2) One Arm Dumbbell Rows – 1 warm up set – 3 sets of 68

3) Seated Rear Delt Flys – 3 sets 68

4) Wide Grip Pull-Downs – 3 sets of 68

5) Standing Barbell Curls – 3 sets of 8

6) Dumbbell Hammer Curls – 2 sets of 8 each arm

Day 3 – Legs and Abs

Walk and Warm Up (Same as Day 1)

1) Bicycle Crunches – 3 sets of 2530

2) V Crunches – 3 sets of 15

3) Leg Press – 12 warm up sets – 4 sets of 8

4) Lying Hamstring Curls – 1 warm up set – 4 sets of 68

5) Standing Lunges with Dumbbells – 4 sets of 8 each leg

6) Standing Calf Raises – 4 sets of 8

Cardio:

Warm up on Bike for 2 minutes then pedal as fast as possible for 20 seconds followed by 1 minute of rest repeat 8 times

OR

Heavy Kettlebell Swings for 20 seconds rest for 20 seconds and repeat 8 times through

OR

Battle Ropes for 20 seconds rest for 20 seconds and repeat 8 times

Day 4 – Chest Shoulders Triceps

Bike or Walk on Treadmill for 5 minutes to break a small sweat

Warm Up: Here is a video that I want you to watch and use to warm up each day

1) Flat Dumbbell Bench Press – 2 warm up sets – 3 sets of 68

2) Standing Dumbbell Shoulder Press – 2 warm up sets – 3 sets of 68

3) Incline Dumbbell Press – 3 sets of 68

4) Standing Side Laterals with Dumbbells – 3 sets of 8

5) Parallel Bar Dips (add weight if necessary) – 2 sets of 68

6) Close Grip Bench Press – 3 sets of 68

7) Captain Chair Leg Raises – 3 sets of 1215

Cardio Workout (can be performed in the morning or evening): 30 minutes steady pace on stepmill, treadmill or elliptical

Day 5 – Back Biceps Rear Delts

Walk and Warm Up (same as Day 1)

1) Wide Grip Pull-Ups – 4 sets of 68 (add weight if necessary)

2) Bent Over Barbell Rows, or T-Bar Rows – 1 warm up set –
   3 sets of 6-8

3) Seated Rear Delt Flys – 3 sets 6-8

4) Seated Cable Rows – 3 sets of 68

5) Standing Dumbbell Curls – 3 sets of 8 each arm

6) Rear Delt Machine Flys – 2 sets of 8

Day 6 – Mix of Cardio

Warm up (Same as Day 1)

Perform the following in a circuit fashion with no rest after
completing all 4 exercises rest for 2 minutes then repeat for 8 rounds.

1) Burpees – 10 reps

2) Medicine Ball Slams – 10 reps

3) Squat Jumps – 10 reps

4) T Push-Ups – 20 reps

Day 7 – Rest

HOTEL WORKOUTS – PICK ONE EACH DAY
WHILE TRAVELING!

Pick up these bands on Amazon. Here I'd suggest starting with the
less resistance (red, black and green).

#**1**

- Every minute on the minute for 1530 minutes (this one will challenge you!)
  - 5 Burpees
  - 10 Push-Ups
  - 15 Jump Squats (odd min do Squats, even min do Jump Squats)

if you do not complete a round in a minute, rest the next minute then resume

#**2**

- Complete 100 Sit-Ups for time

- Rest 2 minutes

- Climb the ladder as high as possible in 12 minutes:

- 3 Hand Release Push-Ups

- 3 Mountain Climbers each leg

- 6 Hand Release Push-Ups

- 6 Mountain Climbers each leg

keep going in increments of 3 until you hit the 12-minute cap

- Rest 2 minutes

- Complete 100 Sit-Ups for time

#**3**

- Jumping Jacks for 5 minutes

- 4 rounds:
  - 25 Bodyweight Squats with bands
  - 12 Lunges each leg
  - 12 Exercise Band Rows
  - 15 Chest Presses with bands

- Rest 5 minutes

For Time:

- 50 Burpees

- 100 Crunches on Exercise Ball

- 200 Mountain Climbers

Cardio While Traveling: 2 sessions of 30 minutes on the Treadmill walking at a decent pace (3.5-4 mph)

CASE STUDY #5: DARYL SPRABARY

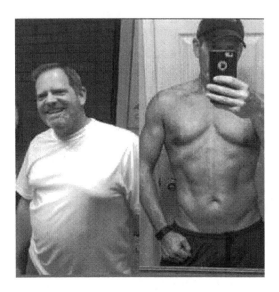

Daryl came to me looking to lose weight. He was worried that his health was suffering big time and he needed a coach to guide him on the best path to get to his goals. As you can see from his pic here – he accomplished more than he ever thought possible!!

Lifestyle Concerns

Daryl's 3 boys were grown and moved out, so he had more flexibility than years past while raising his kids. This gave him more free time to ensure he was getting food prepped and gym sessions complete. His biggest concern was making sure he had the accountability and direction from me, so we set up a consistent check in schedule for him.

Daryl's Meal Plan (in his own words):

Each day is mostly the same, though I intermittent fast about
3 days per week with my first meal at lunch. Learned this from you.
When I do have breakfast, I have oatmeal with some nuts and fruit.
For lunch, I will have chicken breast and a veggie. Save carbs for
dinner. Dinner may be chicken, grain fed beef or bison, lean pork
chop, steak, salmon. Veggies are broccoli, asparagus, sweet potato,
cauliflower rice. I have yet to venture into some of your recipes.
Consistency works well for me. I love good food, but I now eat to live
instead of living to eat.

Daryl's Workout Set-Up (in his own words):

I currently work out 3-4x per week in the evening after dinner
following the challenges you create and or the training app. I've tried
the morning but I'm more effective later in the day.

I usually do 30 min intervals 1-2x per week. Other than that, I walk
when I have the time. I started jumping rope and I do enjoy it,
but I need to find a better rope. I've tried different brands but
haven't found one I love.

Biggest Lessons Daryl learned:

The biggest lessons while working with you has to be diet flexibility
while hitting your macros. I've made the most progress following
detailed plans. Full body workouts are more effective than having
a specific day for a muscle group. We all fail while on this journey as
no one is perfect. Get back up and carry on. Be consistent 80-90%.
I also like the fact that you are a real person. Straight up no bull

shit. I'm that way as well. Always told my kids I would always shoot straight with them and not sugar coat things. That worked well.

CASE STUDY #6: LINDSAY WHEELER

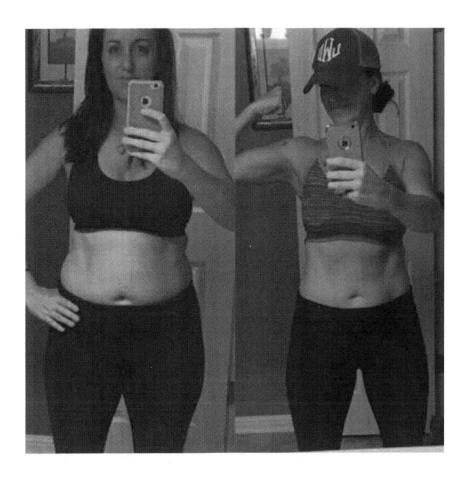

Lindsay is one of the best clients I've ever worked with. She truly changed her entire approach to fitness while working with me and it was in incredible thing to witness. Lindsay came to me feeling pretty down about where she was with her health and fitness goals. As a busy mom, full-time nurse and incredible wife her schedule was jam packed. She had left very little time for herself, but she knew that she'd have to create the time if she was going to make a lasting change.

Lindsay didn't shy away from working hard while going through my programs. Initially she was skeptical for sure, but after giving it a fair shot she realized that this was the program and coaching she had been looking for all along.

Lifestyle Factors:

Lindsay's full-time gig as a nurse meant that she was on her feet a lot and could be susceptible to appetite swings and hunger issues. I made sure to encourage her to have healthy options readily available so that she wasn't grabbing whatever she could find. We also made sure that her plan was set up to keep weekends relatively free for sporting events with her kids and time with her husband and friends.

When I asked her about her lifestyle here's what she said:

> My lifestyle is constantly on the go. I've got 2 boys who are involved in sports. That's 7 practices and 2 games every week between the two of them so I'm constantly running them everywhere. I work 12 hour shifts as a nurse and head committees there too, I'm going to school full time, I volunteer for both kids' PTA, squeeze in dates with my husband and girl time with my friends. Throw in 5 workouts a week, meal prepping, and cleaning the house and you've got my life!

NUTRITION Plan (in her own words):

My typical meal plan really is enjoying the foods I love and throwing a healthy twist on them. I use My Fitness Pal to manage my macros.

I meal prep 1-2 times a week which helps keep me on track. I try not to stress about food too much because I don't want to create an aversion to eating healthy. I keep it simple and add spices to make it interesting. I typically Intermittent fast most days. I'll have a protein shake, maybe some ground turkey with rice and a veggie, and a dinner that's on the healthy side. I'll switch up my meal preps, so I don't get bored.

Workout Plan for Lindsay:

Day 1: Full Body Workout

Day 2: Cardio 20 minutes

Day 3: OFF

Day 4: Full Body Workouts

Day 5: Cardio

Day 6: Light Activity

Day 7: OFF

Day 1 – Full Body Weights

Warm Up: 5-10 minutes on bike

1) Dynamic Stretching for 5 minutes

2) Rest Between Sets: 60-90 seconds

3) Standing Squats to Push Press with Dumbbells – 4 sets of 10-12

4) Push-Ups on Knees – 3 sets of 10-12

5) Standing Lunges with Dumbbell Curls (curl both arms at same time) after each lunge – 4 sets of 10-12

6) Bent Over One Arm Rows with Dumbbells or Heavy Object – 3 sets of 10-12

7) Overhead Tricep Dumbbell Extensions – 2 sets of 10-12

8) Crunches – 3 sets of 15-20

Day 2 – Walk or Bike for 20 minutes

Day 3 – OFF

Day 4 – Full Body Weights

Warm Up: 5-10 minutes on bike

1) Dynamic Stretching for 5 minutes

2) Rest Between Sets: 60-90 seconds

3) Standing Squats to Push Press with Dumbbells – 4 sets of 10-12

4) Push-Ups on Knees – 3 sets of 10-12

5) Standing Lunges with Dumbbell Curls (curl both arms at same time) after each lunge – 4 sets of 10-12

6) Bent Over One Arm Rows with Dumbbells or Heavy Object – 3 sets of 10-12

7) Overhead Tricep Dumbbell Extensions – 2 sets of 10-12

8) Crunches – 3 sets of 15-20

Day 5 – 20 minutes of cardio

Day 6 – Bike or Walk for 20 minutes and/or YOGA

Day 7 – OFF

Lindsay's Results (in her own words):

My results have blown me away!! At 39, I feel the best I've felt since I was 20! I'm actually in better shape than I was then! I've lost 30 lbs. and have kept it off. I have muscles that you can actually see which is fun!! And the best part is that my kids and husband are proud of the hard work and dedication they've seen me invest in myself. I have more energy, self-awareness, and drive than I did before too!

CASE STUDY #7: TONY LASICA

When I first started working with Tony he was very frustrated. He had done CrossFit and then hired another online coach who ended up not working well for him. His goal was simple – he wanted to lose belly-fat and see his abs. Little did we know that this would turn into something even bigger.

Tony followed everything I told him to do. And his results were absolutely insane. He got lean, more muscular and his love for fitness skyrocketed. He had finally cracked the code to achieving his all-time best physique. His new-found passion for getting lean drove him to do something he'd never even thought of doing before – entering a physique competition.

Long story short he dieted down to extremely low levels of body-fat and ended up placing top 3 in his first show. Tony being the competitive person that he is, decided that he wanted to try for another show and win this time. So, after a few months of relaxation and bringing his calories back up we picked another a 2nd show target. Despite a pretty tough prep, Tony wound up winning his class at his 2nd show!

Tony, besides having a killer work ethic, is married, has 2 amazing kids and works his ass off in the medical industry. This guy is a true example of hard work, trusting the process and consistency can do. Here's how he described his lifestyle:

Typical life of a married man with school aged kids. My work days are usually about 14 hrs., I leave the house at 0530 am and usually get home around 8 pm. My wife works a similar schedule. I don't have a job where I can work out during lunch, and those few hours of precious family time we have at night can't be spent with me in the gym. Evenings are usually occupied by the kid's sports schedules. This doesn't leave me with much "free" time to work out, this isn't something I do in my spare time, or out of convenience. Making this a priority means me often setting my alarm for 330 am in order to make time for the gym on a consistent basis. Looking and feeling a certain way is why I do this, and Josiah has shown me how to achieve my goals – but it requires me making it a priority each and every day.

The biggest lessons he learned while working with me (in his own words):

Consistency is king. Trying to be perfect isn't sustainable and will result in failure eventually. Developing a solid foundation of good habits is the key to making this work for the long haul. There's a ton of motivation early on during a transformation – but eventually those motivating factors level out, and you have to be able to fall back on something to continue having success.

Tony's Nutrition Game plan (in his own words):

My diet has been of the balanced variety with a pretty heavy lean on carbohydrates, utilizing intermittent fasting daily.

Tony's Starting Workout Plan:

PHASE 1: FOUNDATIONS

- Goal: Strength, Muscle Density, and Power. Each week you should be aiming to get stronger on all exercises.

- Length: 4 Weeks

Rest Time in Between Sets: 2-3 minutes

Day 1 – Upper Focus (Bench Strength)

Dynamic Warm Up

1) Activation: Hand Release Push-Ups – 2 sets of 6-8

2) Bench Press
   - Week 1: 3 sets of 5
   - Week 2: 4 sets of 4
   - Week 3: 5 sets of 2
   - Week 4: 3 sets of 5 (re-test from week 1)

3) Pendley Row or Seal Rows – 4 sets of 4-6 reps

4) Standing Dumbbell Press – 3 sets of 4-6 reps

5) Pull-Ups – 3 sets of 4-6 reps

6) Weighted Hanging Leg Raises – 3 sets of 8-10

Day 2 – Lower Body Focus

Warm Up

1) Activation: High Jumps – 2 sets of 6-8

2) Squats
   - Week 1: 3 sets of 5
   - Week 2: 4 sets of 4
   - Week 3: 5 sets of 2
   - Week 4: 3 sets of 5 (re-test from week 1)

3) Romanian Deadlifts – 3 sets of 6

4) Box Step-Ups – 3 sets of 5 each leg

Day 3:

1) Exercise Band Circuits (Active Recovery)

2) 3 x per day set aside 10 minutes to complete as many rounds of the following circuit as possible.
   - 10 Push-Ups
   - 10 Exercise Band Rows
   - 10 Exercise Band Side Laterals
   - 10 Exercise Bands Curls
   - 10 Exercise Band Tricep Overhead Extensions
   - 10 Crunches

Day 4 – Upper Focus (Standing Overhead Press Strength)

Warm Up

1) Activate: 2 sets of Side Laterals (8-10 reps)

2) Standing Overhead Press
   - Week 1: 3 sets of 5
   - Week 2: 4 sets of 4
   - Week 3: 5 sets of 2
   - Week 4: 3 sets of 5 (re-test from week 1)

3) Incline Bench 2 Arm Dumbbell Rows – 3 sets of 3-6

4) Incline Dumbbell Press – 3 sets of 3-6

5) Rear Delt Machine Flys – 2 sets of 6-8

6) Barbell Curls – 2 sets of 4-6

7) Skullcrushers – 2 sets of 4-6

Day 5 – Lower Body Focus (Deadlift Day)

Warm Up

1) Activate: Long Jumps – 2 sets of 4

2) Deadlifts:
   - Week 1: 3 sets of 5
   - Week 2: 4 sets of 4
   - Week 3: 5 sets of 2
   - Week 4: 3 sets of 5 (re-test from week 1)

3) Front Squats – 3 sets of 4-6

4) Lying Leg Curls – 3 sets of 6

5) Standing Calf Raises – 3 sets of 6-8

6) Weighted Decline Crunches – 3 sets of 10

Tony's Results (in his own words):

In January of 2017 I weighed about 185 lbs., with a body fat percentage somewhere in the mid 20's. Since May of 2017 I've weighed between 155-160 consistently, maintaining a body fat percentage of about 8-10%. I've done 2 physique shows in that time dropping down to below 150 lbs. and a body fat percentage of around 6. The results achieved go way beyond just numbers – the confidence and energy that has come with it is what has been the most gratifying.

CASE STUDY #8: JASON DURANT

Jason has lost over 100 lbs. while working with me!! This guy has been the definition of hard work while working with me. His career puts him in high heat most of the day and he's had to find the drive and willpower to hit the gym early in the day or during his lunch break which isn't easy to do when you're on your feet for 12 hours a day!

Jason is an example of what's possible if you invest in yourself and never look back. I can't say enough about how proud of I am of Jason and the transformation he's made.

Lifestyle Considerations:

For Jason the main things we focused on were giving him enough flexibility with his nutrition without setting him up for failure. He tracked his calories which allowed him to fit in some "bad" foods here and there but for the most part he stuck with healthy options that kept his appetite and energy stable.

I asked Jason to describe working with me and here's what he had to say:

> So, working with you I can say that my biggest lesson learned is that I don't have to eat nothing but chicken and veggies to lose weight. I also learned that the typical weight program of doing one muscle group a day is boring! I love the total body workouts and the upper/lower splits. I have been able to fit my workouts in without compromising time with my work or my family time. I generally workout at 330am before I get ready for work. My meal plan has always been to make sure I hit my macros regardless of the food I eat. No chicken and veggies every day. I learned to live my life and enjoy food at the same time I was losing over

100 pounds! And keep it off even when I'm busy and had to put workouts on hold for a while. I started out with 5 days a week of working out now it's 3 to 4 depending on my schedule. I never do cardio unless I feel like running which I did for a while, but I get my heart rate raised the same with lifting and metabolic cardio and get more benefits than I did just running on the hamster wheel! I went from a 286 lb heart-attack walking to a 173 lb, healthy 40-year-old. I've added some muscle to my frame and now weigh between 180-185 and feel amazing.

Incredible!!

Jason's Workout Plan:

Each week we will dedicate 2 days to building strength one for upper body and one for lower body. The other 3 days will be more geared towards muscle size and burning calories. We will train each muscle group 2x per week.

I only want you pushing to failure on your last set of each exercise. All other sets should be stopped about 12 reps before failure. This ensures that your Central Nervous System is kept in good shape.

Cardio will be 3 sessions per week. One session can be something like walking on the treadmill, the elliptical or step mill for 30 minutes. One session will be a quick 10-minute High Intensity session and the last session will be a mix of both. You can also do things like swimming, biking or hiking for your first 30-minute session.

Each week I want you to try and beat the previous weeks numbers by adding either 12 reps or adding 5 lbs to your sets and getting the same reps.

Day 1 – Upper Strength

Bike or Walk on Treadmill for 5 minutes to break a small sweat

Warm Up: Here is a video that I want you to watch and use to warm up each day.

1) Pull-Ups – 3 sets of 58

2) OneArm Dumbbell Row – 1 warm up set – 3 sets of 48 each arm

3) Flat Bench Press – 2 warm up sets – 3 sets of 46

4) Seated Shoulder Dumbbell Press – 12 warm up sets – 3 sets 68

5) Parallel Bar Dips – 2 sets of 6

6) Standing Barbell Curls – 2 sets of 68

Cardio: 30 minutes steady pace

Day 2 – Lower Strength

Walk and Warm Up (Same as Day 1)

1) Leg Press – 2 warm up sets – 3 sets of 68

2) Lying Leg Curls – 2 warm up sets – 3 sets of 68

3) Hack Squat – 3 sets 68

4) Lunges with Dumbbells or Leg Extensions – 2 sets of 68

Day 3 – Chest and Arms

Walk and Warm Up (Same as Day 1)

1) Bicycle Crunches – 3 sets of 2530

2) V Crunches – 3 sets of 15

3) Incline Dumbbell Press – 12 warm up sets – 4 sets of 1215

4) Flat Dumbbell Flys – 4 sets of 1215

5) Standing Dumbbell Curls – 1 warm up set – 4 sets of 10 each arm

6) Tricep Rope Push-Downs

7) Jump Squats – 2 sets of 8 – 4 sets of 1215

8) Hammer Curls – 2 sets of 10 each arm

Cardio: Warm up on Bike for 2 minutes then pedal as fast as possible for 20 seconds followed by 1 minute of rest repeat 8 times

Day 4 – Legs

Walk and Warm Up (Same as Day 1)

1) Lying Leg Curls – 3 sets of 15

2) Leg Extensions – 3 sets of 15

3) Sumo Deadlifts – 3 sets of 10

4) Standing Calf Raises – 3 sets of 15

5) Crunches on Stability Ball – 3 sets of 20

Day 5 – Back and Shoulders

1) Wide Grip Lat Pulldown – 3 sets of 1215

2) Seated Rows – 3 sets of 1215

3) Standing Side Laterals – 3 sets of 1215

4) Rear Delt Machine Flys – 3 sets of 1215

5) Underhand Pull-Downs – 3 sets of 1215

Day 6 – Mix of Cardio

Warm up (Same as Day 1)

Perform the following in a circuit fashion with no rest after completing all 4 exercises rest for 2 minutes then repeat for 5 rounds.

1) Burpees – 10 reps

2) Medicine Ball Slams – 10 reps

3) Squat Jumps – 10 reps

4) T Push-Ups – 20 reps

After 5 rounds complete 20 minutes of moderate pace cardio on your choice of equipment.

Made in the USA
Middletown, DE
15 November 2018